Narjes ABID
Sameh MSAAD

59 cases of occupational asthma

Narjes ABID
Sameh MSAAD

59 cases of occupational asthma

ScienciaScripts

Imprint
Any brand names and product names mentioned in this book are subject to trademark, brand or patent protection and are trademarks or registered trademarks of their respective holders. The use of brand names, product names, common names, trade names, product descriptions etc. even without a particular marking in this work is in no way to be construed to mean that such names may be regarded as unrestricted in respect of trademark and brand protection legislation and could thus be used by anyone.

Cover image: www.ingimage.com

This book is a translation from the original published under ISBN 978-620-6-72331-8.

Publisher:
Sciencia Scripts
is a trademark of
Dodo Books Indian Ocean Ltd. and OmniScriptum S.R.L publishing group

120 High Road, East Finchley, London, N2 9ED, United Kingdom
Str. Armeneasca 28/1, office 1, Chisinau MD-2012, Republic of Moldova, Europe
Printed at: see last page
ISBN: 978-620-8-34069-8

Copyright © Narjes ABID, Sameh MSAAD
Copyright © 2024 Dodo Books Indian Ocean Ltd. and OmniScriptum S.R.L publishing group

Contents

A

My dear Father Nouri

To whom I owe everything

You've devoted your whole life to looking after our family.

It is your *constant support, your boundless sacrifices sacrifices, your availability and generosity that have allowed me to be what I am today.*

May you find in this work the expression of my deepest gratitude.

"may god preserve you for us and grant you good health

long life and happiness".

A

My dear mother Monjia

You've done more than any mother can do to ensure that

her children follow the right path in their lives and their studies.

Your prayers and blessings have been a great help to

me in my studies.

I dedicate this work to you as a token of my deep gratitude.

"may god preserve you for us and grant you good

health
long life and happiness".

A

My dear husband Karim

NuUe dedicate cannot express my love and
deep affection.
Even on the other side of the world, you've always been
there
for me.
Without your help, advice and encouragement, this
work would never have seen the light of day.
Thank you for giving meaning to my life
Thank you for being ld for me
Special dedication to you
"May god keep us united and happy".

A

My dear twin sister Naoures

You are not just a sister to me, but my soul
sister and my best friend
We have shared many pleasant moments and
we have always helped each other during our long
course of study.
I dedicate this work to you as a token of my deep
affection
"May God protect you and give you a pleasant life
full of joy and happiness".

My dear brother Bassem and his wife Mariem

My dear brother, who has always helped me, who has been
where and when I needed him.
I dedicate this work to you both as a token of
my deep affection.
"May God protect you and preserve your health,
happiness and success".

My grandparents Hssan and Jamila
The memory of my grandparents
Sadok and Majida

A

My parents-in-law Taoufik and Samira

A

My brothers-in-law

Imed and his wife Asma

HiChem and his wife Najta

Slim and his wife Samira

Hassen and his fiancée Sahar

To the little angels

Sana, Nada

Mahdi, Mohamed Amine

Yassine, Mahmoud

To all families
Abid
Bejar
Samet

A

All my friends

A

All medical and paramedical staff in the departments

PneumOogie EPS Hed Cheker, Sfax
Internal Medicine EPS Hedi Cheker, Sfax Infectious Diseases EPS Hedi Cheker, Sfax
Chirurgie Generale EPS Habib Bourguiba, Sfax
Oto- rhino- laryngologie EPS Habib Bourguiba, Sfax
Gynecology I'hopital regional de Djbeniana
Pediatrics EPS Hedi Cheker, Sfax
Preventive medicine EPS Hedi Cheker, Sfax

Our Master and President of the jury Professor Abdelkader Ayoub

Head of Pneumology Department

, Hedi Chaker University Hospital, Sfax

You are doing us the great honour of chairing the jury for this thesis.

Your skill and dedication are an example to us all.

I would like to express my sincere gratitude for your teaching and guidance

Please find in this work *the* expression of *our* deep gratitude

Our Master and judge and director of these Professor

Samya Marouen Jamoussi

Occupational Medicine Department

At the Hedi Chaker University Hospital in Sfax

I am grateful to you for directing this work.

Your competence, dedication and extreme kindness kindness really impressed us and are an example to us all.

I would like to express my deep gratitude to you for this work.

Our Master and judge of these Professor Agrege Wajdi Karim Rekik

Pneumology Department

At the Hedi Chaker University Hospital in Sfax

I would like to thank you very much, dear master, for the honour
for the honour you have done me by agreeing to be the jury of this thesis
Please find in this work the expression of my deep respect
respect for your human, scientific and professional scientific and professional qualities

Our Master and Judge of these Professor Agrége

Hajeur Ayedi

Pneumology Department

, CHU Hedi Chaker, Sfax

I would like to thank you most sincerely for the great honour

you have done me by agreeing to judge this work.

I admire your wealth of knowledge and your scientific rigour

Please accept my warm thanks and

deep respect

Our Master and Judge of these

, Professor

Ben Ayed Mourad

Functional exploration department

at the Habib Bourguiba University Hospital in Sfax

I would like to thank you most sincerely for the great honour

you have done me by agreeing to judge this work.

Please find in this work

the expression of my deepest respect.

Our Master and thesis director
Dear Doctor
Msaad Sameh

University Hospital Assistant in the Pneumology Department
At the Hedi Chaker University Hospital in Sfax
I am grateful to you for directing this work.
Your scientific and human qualities and your professional dynamism
dynamism are an example to me.
Your contribution to my training and
Your sense of efficiency command my admiration
Please find in this work a modest token of my deepest respect and my sincere thanks.

Our Master
Dear Professor
Samy Kammoun

Professor in the Pneumology Department
at the Hedi Chaker University Hospital in Sfax
Your skills and your scientific and human qualities
are an example to us all
Through this work, I would like to express my deep esteem and sincere gratitude.

Our Master

, Professor

Ilhem Yengui

Pneumology Department

At the Hedi Chaker University Hospital in Sfax

Your dedication, your knowledge and your human qualities

human qualities have always impressed us

Please find in this work the expression of my respect

respect and my profound gratitude

Our Master

Dear Doctor

Wajdi Ketata

University Hospital Assistant in the Pneumology Department at the Hedi Chaker University Hospital in Sfax

We appreciate your great modesty, your human qualities and

and your scientific rigour.

Please find in this work the expression of *my deep esteem*

قسم الطبيب

اقسم بالله العظيم

- أن أراقب الله في مهنتي.
- وأن أصون حياة الإنسان في كافة أدوارها، في كل الظروف والأحوال باذلا وسعي في استنقاذها من الهلاك والمرض والألم والقلق.
- وأن أحفظ للناس كرامتهم، وأستر عورتهم، وأكتم سرهم.
- وأن أكون على الدوام من وسائل رحمة الله، باذلا رعايتي الطبيّة للقريب والبعيد، للصالح والخاطئ، والصديق والعدو.
- وأن أثابر على طلب العلم، أسخره لنفع الإنسان لا لأذاه.
- وأن أوقّر من علّمني، وأعلم من يصغرني، وأكون أخا لكلّ زميل في المهنة الطبيّة متعاونين على البر والتقوى.
- وأن تكون حياتي مصداق إيماني في سرّي و علا نيتي، نقية ممّا يشينها تجاه الله ورسوله والمؤمنين.

والله على ما أقول شهيد

HIPPOCRATIC OATH

In the presence of the masters of this school, my dear fellow students and in the tradition of Hippocrates, I promise and swear to be faithful to the ois of honour and probity in the practice of medicine.

I would give Cindigent my free care and would never demand a salary above my work.

If I go inside a house, my eyes won't see what's going on there.

My tongue will keep silent about the secrets entrusted to me, and my state will not be used to corrupt morals or encourage crime.

Respectful and grateful to my teachers, I will give back to their children the same education I received from their fathers.

May men esteem me if I am faithful to my promises, and may I be shamed and despised by my colleagues if I fail to keep them.

1 INTRODUCTION

Many workers inhale contaminants of various types in the general environment and in the workplace. These contaminants can damage the respiratory system and contribute to the emergence of occupational lung diseases (OLD), including asthma.

Ramazzini, in 1700, was one of the first to describe certain cases of occupational asthma (OA), particularly among millers.

PA, which affects economically active subjects, currently appears to be the most common occupational respiratory disease [1, 2, 3, 4]. This is due to the ever-increasing number of new potentially hazardous substances being introduced into industry.

However, the incidence of PA remains underestimated due to diagnostic difficulties, the large number of causative agents and the under-reporting of this disease by doctors and employees. [3]

Diagnosis of this disease requires an appropriate approach, combining careful questioning with a functional respiratory and immunological work-up, with three main objectives: to establish a positive diagnosis of asthma; to demonstrate the occupational origin of the disease; and to identify the causative agent [5].

The social repercussions of PA are major. Its economic consequences, due to the direct cost of the disease itself, its treatment, absenteeism and loss of professional efficiency, are of paramount importance.

In this study, we were interested in cases of asthma declared as an occupational disease, with the following objectives:

- ❖ Study the frequency of PA in southern Tunisia from 2002 to 2009.
- ❖ To determine the diagnostic strategy for PA and the epidemiological characteristics of the subjects affected.
- ❖ Describe the etiological factors, in particular the main professions involved.
- ❖ Describe the therapeutic, evolutionary and preventive aspects, and the medical-legal reparation.

2 MATERIALS AND METHODS

1. Type of study

This is a retrospective descriptive study conducted in the Occupational Medicine and Pathology Department of the Hedi Cheker University Hospital, Sfax, in collaboration with the Pneumology Department and the regional offices of the National Health Insurance Fund (CNAM).

2. Study population

Our survey covered all the PA cases reported to the CNAM regional offices over an eight-year period from 01/01/2002 to 31/12/2009.

3. Data collection

We consulted :

❖ Patient files are filed in the Pneumology Department archives.

❖ The medical and administrative records of patients declared under the PA (initial medical certificate (CMI), para-clinical assessment, etc.) collected from the CNAM regional offices in Sfax.

❖ Data from the occupational survey carried out by THE CNAM for all declared cases.

The data collected is recorded on a synoptic sheet containing a number of headings:

1) The patient's identity (surname, first name, age, sex)
2) Socio-professional data

❖ Geographical origin

❖ Marital status

❖ School level

❖ Type of social security scheme

❖ Work sector

❖ Profession(s)

❖ Professional category

❖ Date of hire

❖ Data from the workstation study

3) The patient's personal and family medical antecedents and habits.
4) The history and clinical examination.
5) Results of practical supplementary examinations :

❖ Biological tests (NFS, total and specific IgE)

❖ Radiological check-up (chest and sinus X-rays)

❖ RESPIRATORY function tests (Spirometry, simple and stepwise, specific and non-specific bronchial provocation test, reversibility test to mimetic B2, eviction test)

❖ Allergological skin tests (standard and specific prick tests)

6) Therapeutic and developmental approaches.
7) Medical and legal consequences.

The various data will be summarised in the results section.

It is important to specify that the inclusion criteria for asthma cases are :

1) All patients with a professional activity and of professional age declared as PA.

2) The diagnosis of asthma is confirmed by a lung specialist and/or a doctor specialising in occupational pathology on the basis of :

❖ A clinical history suggestive of asthma

❖ Lung function tests compatible with a diagnosis of bronchial asthma.

3) All cases of asthma declared as an occupational disease and discussed by the specialist occupational disease recognition committee.

Not included:

1) All cases of asthma diagnosed in patients who do not have a professional activity declared to the CNAM.
2) All cases of allergic rhinitis without associated obstructive syndrome.

4. Definitions

- <u>Obstructive ventilatory disorder</u>: is defined by a Tiffenau ratio of less than 0.7. The severity of the OVD is judged by the FEV1 value. OVD is therefore :
- Mild if FEV1 > 80
- Moderate if FEV1 is between [60-80%].
- Severe if FEV1 between [30- 60%[.
- Very severe if FEV1 < 30%.
- <u>Non-specific bronchial hyperreactivity</u> (NSABH) is defined as excessive bronchial obstruction in response to various stimuli that produce little or no response in normal individuals.

To test for HRBNS, a quantitative test is used, in which increasing doses of metacholine or carbachol are administered in aerosol form, starting at 50 ug. After each dose, FEV1 is measured. A decrease in FEV1 of more than 20% is required for a dose of less than 3000 ug to be considered a positive test.

5. Interpretation criteria for biological tests *and immunological*

❖ The eosinophil count is considered high (hyper eosinophilia) from 400 El/ml).

❖ Total Ig E levels are considered high from 100IU/1

6. Statistical analysis

For statistical analysis, the data were entered and analysed using SPSS version 18.0 software.

Correlations were studied using a bivariate analysis based on Pearson's correlation coefficient. The correlation is stronger if the value is close to -1 or 1. Significance is acquired for a $p < 0.05$ for all statistical tests.

3 RESULTS

Between 01/01/2002 and 31/12/2009, we were able to identify 59 cases of PA among 686 cases of occupational disease (OD) declared at the various CNAM regional offices in southern Tunisia, i.e. 8.6% of all OD declared.

1. Breakdown of HA cases by year of notification

The breakdown of cases by year of notification was as follows (Figure 1):

- In 2002: 7 cases, or 11.8% of all cases.
- In 2003: 8 cases, or 13.5% of all cases.
- In 2004: 12 cases, or 20.3% of all cases.
- In 2005: 9 cases, or 15.2% of all cases.
- In 2006: 10 cases, or 16.9% of all cases.
- In 2007: 8 cases, or 13.5% of all cases.
- In 2008: 4 cases, or 6.7% of all cases.
- In 2009: 1 case, or 1.6% of all cases.

The average number of cases reported per year is 7.3.

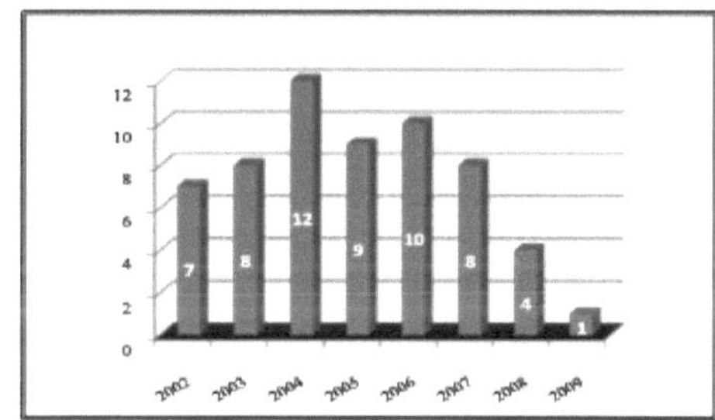

Figure 1: Distribution of HA cases by year of notification

2. Breakdown of reported cases by socio-demographic data

2.1. Gender

Our population is predominantly male (74.5%). The sex ratio is estimated at 2.93 (Figure 2).

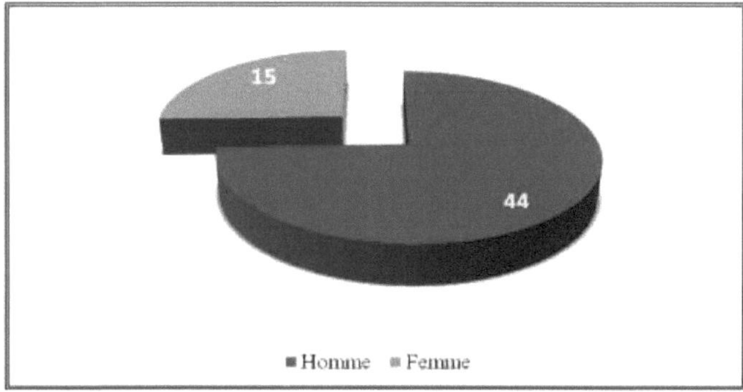

Figure 2: Breakdown of the population by gender

2.2. Age

The average age of patients was 42 ± 9 years, with extremes ranging from 24 to 64 years (Figure 3).

The average age of the male population is 44. The average age for women is 36.

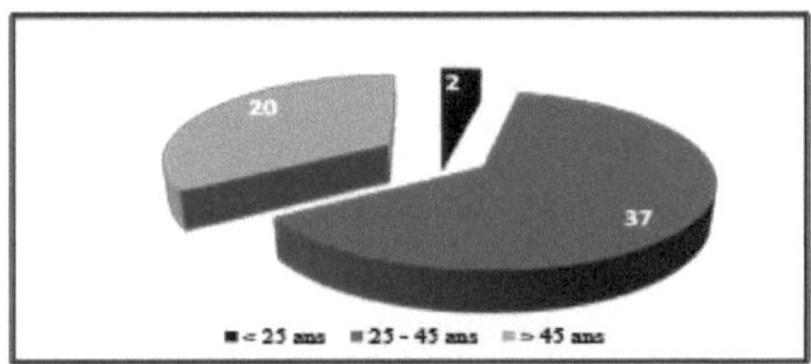

Figure 3: *Age distribution of the population*

All the men were aged over 25 and were almost equally divided between the two age groups [25-45] (24 men or 54.5%) and > 45 (20 men or 45.4%).

The majority of the female population is aged between 25 and 45 (13 women or 18.6%). No woman was aged over 45 (Figure 4).

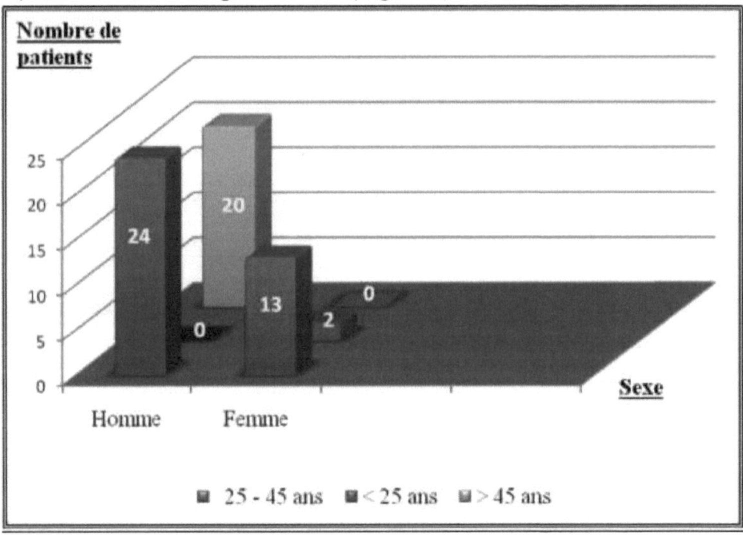

Figure 4 : Breakdown of the population studied by age and gender

2.3. Geographical origin :

More than half the patients were from the town of Sfax (54.2% of cases). The other cases were mainly from Sidi Bouzid (20.3% of cases) and Kasserine (10.1% of cases).

The breakdown of patients by geographical origin is shown in the table and figures below (Table I and Figures 5 and 6).

Table I: Breakdown of patients by geographical origin

Geographical origin	*Number of cases*	*Frequency(%) (N=59)*
Sfax	32	54,2
Sidi Bouzid	12	20,3
Kasserine	6	10,1
Medenine	4	6,7
Gabes	2	3,3
Tataouine	2	3,3
Tozeur	1	1,6

The region of Kasserine, Medenine, Sfax and Sidi Bouzid is characterised by a predominance of male patients (Figure 5).

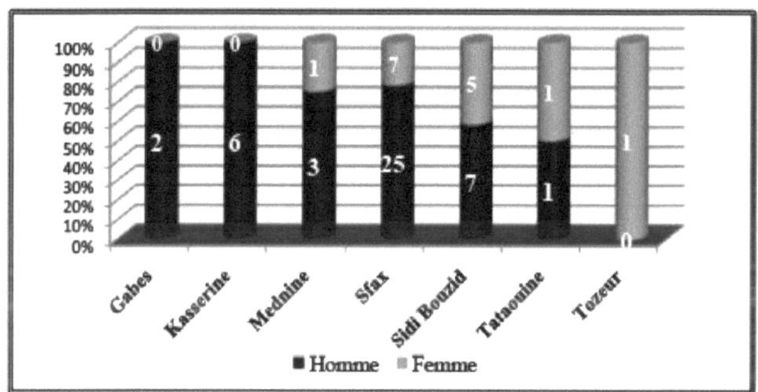

Figure 5 : Breakdown of the population by geographical origin and gender

In the Sfax and Sidi Bouzid regions, most of the population is between 25 and 45 years of age. In Gabes, the two patients reported were aged over 45 (Figure 6).

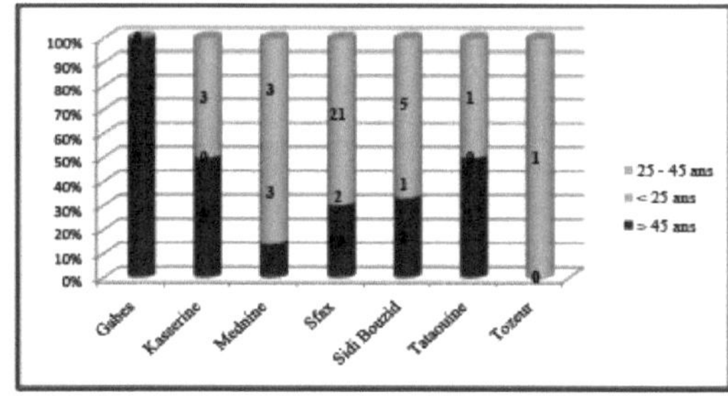

Figure 6: Breakdown of the population by geographical origin and age

3. Professional data

3.1. Sector of activity

The majority of patients (80.3% of cases) work in companies in the secondary sector (manufacturing industry). Only one case was recorded in the primary sector (Figure 7).

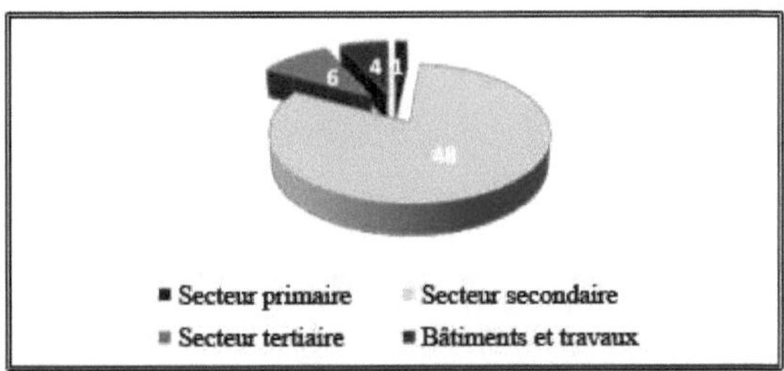

Figure 7: Breakdown of reported cases by economic sector

Within the secondary sector, the most common sectors are: the food industry (28.8%), textiles and clothing (16.9%), the chemical industry (13.5%), carpentry and the wood industry (11.8%) and the metal industry (10.1%) (Table II).

Table II: Breakdown of reported cases by sector of activity

Sector of activity	Domain	Number of patients	Percentage (%) N=59
Primary sector	Industry extractive	1	1,6
	Food industry	17	28,8
	Textiles and clothing	10	16,9
Secondary sector	Chemical industry	8	13,5
	Joinery and industry wood	7	11,8
	Industry metallic	6	10,1
	Health	4	6,7
Tertiary sector	Hotellerie	2	3,3
Buildings and works audiences		4	6,7

3.2. Profession

The twenty skilled workers include five bakers, a pastry chef, two drivers, a seamstress, three carpenters, two painters, a welder, a turner and a varnisher. The two middle managers are a nurse and a senior technician (Figure 8).

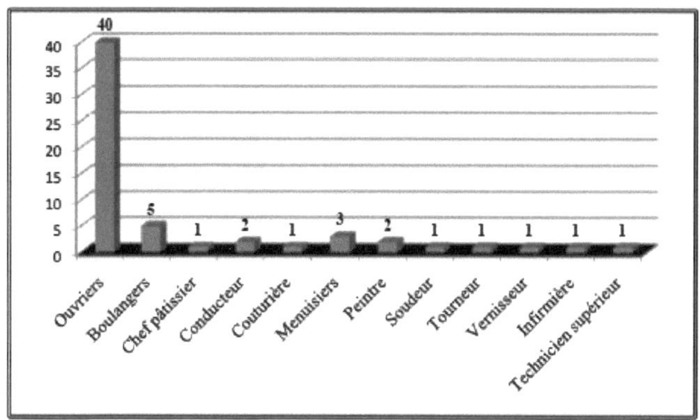

Figure 8: Breakdown of population by occupation

3.3. Professional category

Forty patients belonged to the blue-collar category, representing a majority (67.7%). The other patients included 17 skilled workers (28.8%) and two middle managers (3.3%). There were no senior managers among our patients (Figure 9).

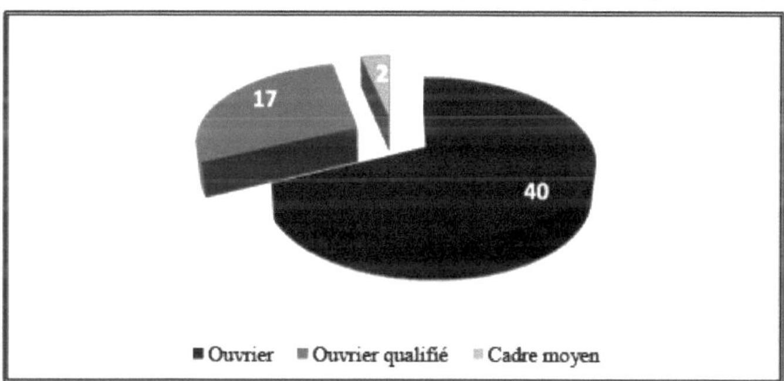

Figure 9: Breakdown of reported cases by occupational category

3.4. Social security cover

All patients belong to the private sector and benefit from health insurance provided by the CNAM.

3.5. Occupational medicine coverage

More than 2/3 of the population (67.7% of cases) are covered by occupational medicine (Figure 10).

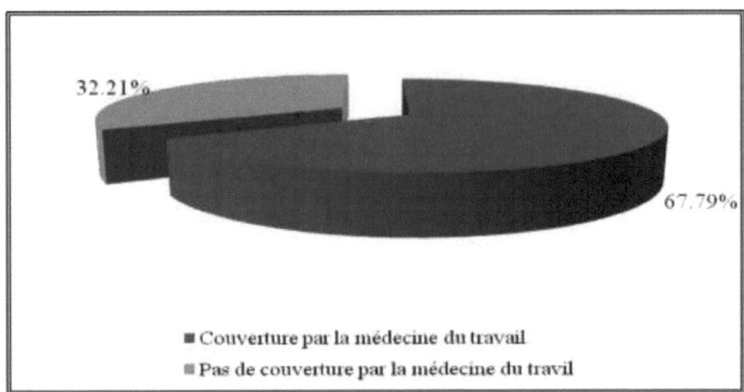

Figure 10: Breakdown of reported cases according to whether or not they were covered by occupational medicine

Almost 80% of patients from Sfax and Sidi Bouzid benefited from this coverage by regional occupational medicine structures (Figure11).

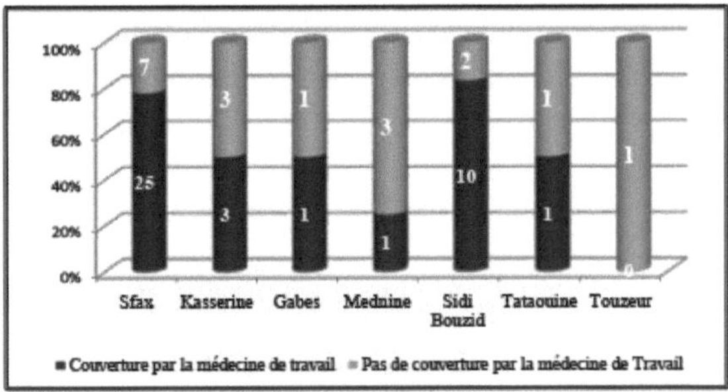

Figure 11: Breakdown of the population studied by geographical origin and occupational health coverage

4. Diagnosis of asthma

4.1. Questioning

4.1.1. Background

❖ Atopic antecedents

Only one patient in our series had a family history of atopy. Personal antecedents of atopy were identified in 13 patients (20.3%). These were :

6 cases of allergic asthma ;

6 cases of allergic rhinitis ;

One case of eczema (Table III).

It should also be noted that the majority of patients (77%) had no history of atopy.

Table III: Frequency of personal atopic antecedents

Personal history of atopy	Number of patients	Frequency (%)
No	46	77,9
Allergic asthma	6	10,1
Allergic rhinitis	6	10,1
Eczema	1	1,6
Allergic conjunctivitis	0	0

❖ Other antecedents

A history of treated and cured common pulmonary tuberculosis was reported in 2 patients.

1.1.2. Reason for consultation :

The majority of patients, 81.3%, had received at least one occupational medicine consultation for suspected occupational disease (Figure 12).

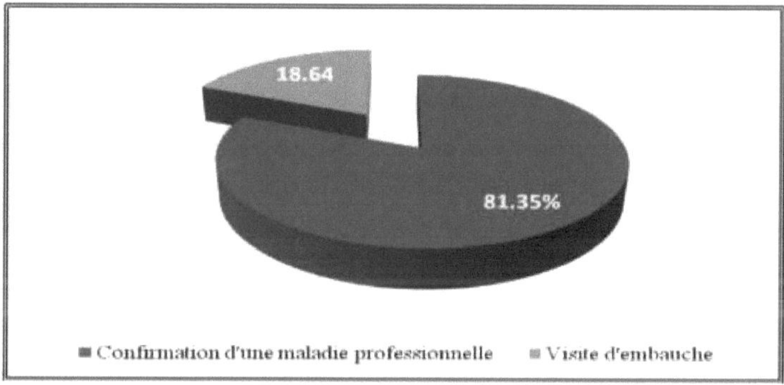

Figure 12: Breakdown of the population studied by reason for consultation

1.1.3. Functional respiratory signs

Forty-four patients reported variable wheezing, which was the main functional complaint in our series (74.5%). Chronic dry cough was noted in 13 patients (22%) (Table VI).

Table VI: Respiratory signs reported by patients

Clinical manifestation	*Number*	*Frequency (%)*
Wheezing dyspnea	44	74,5
Dry cough	13	22
Sneezing	6	10,1
Dyspnea + cough	9	15,2
Atopic manifestations	22	37,2
Dyspnea + atopic symptoms	15	25,4

4.2. Somatic examination

The physical examination was without notable abnormality in almost half the

patients (44%). Wheezing and snoring were noted in 37.2% and 11.8% of patients respectively.
Data from the skin, ear, nose and throat examinations, as well as
and ophthalmology were not specified in our files.

4.3. Paraclinical assessment

4.3.1. Radiological check-up

In all patients, the initial diagnostic work-up included a standard frontal chest X-ray. No significant abnormalities were found except for thoracic distension in 6 cases and bronchial syndrome in 4 others (Table V).

Table V: Distribution of the population according to the data from the standard
chest X-ray

Chest X-ray data standard	*Number of patients*	*Frequency (%)*
Normal	49	83
Chest distension	6	10,1
Bronchial syndrome	4	6,7

In addition, sinus radiography was performed in only 3 patients. This revealed maxillary filling in one case and pansinusitis in the other two.

4.3.2. Biological and immunological tests

Figure 1 Blood count

Of the 10 patients in whom a blood count was performed, 7 (11.8%) had hyper eosinophilia with a blood eosinophil count of over 500 elements/mm3.

Figure 2 Determination of total Ig E

Total Ig E was measured in 18 patients (30.5% of the population). An increased level exceeding 150 IU/ml was found in 11 of the 18 patients who benefited from a total IgE assay, i.e. 61.1% of cases (Figure13).

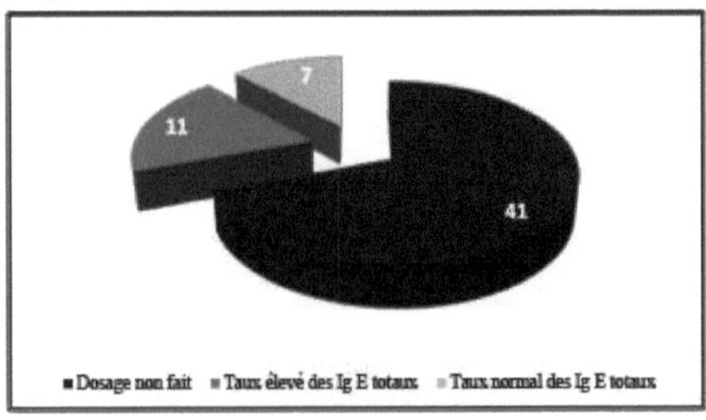

Figure 13 Blood level of total Ig E

❖ Prick test standard

As part of the allergological study, only patients aged under 40 and presenting a clinical picture suggestive of atopy were given a prick test, i.e. 27 patients (45.7%). Sensitisation to one or more allergens was confirmed in 18 cases (66.6%), representing almost a third of the total population (30.5%) (Figure 14).

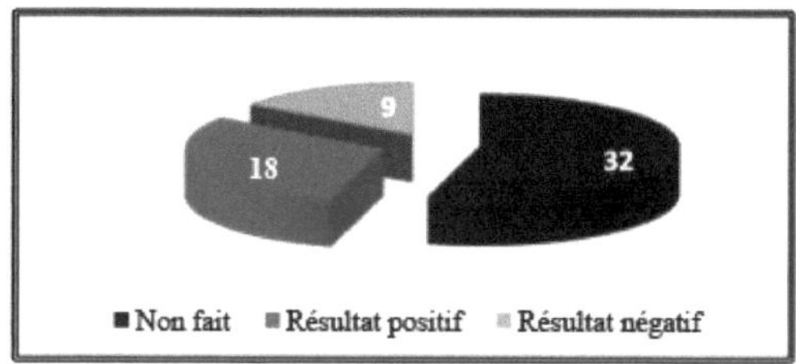

Figure 14 Results of standard prick tests

4.3.3. Respiratory function assessment

❖ Spirometry with flow/volume curve

Spirometry results were not found in 11 cases. The reports were therefore analysed in only 48 patients. Among the cases analysed, the mean value of the FEV1:FVC ratio was 65.6%. Spirometry was normal in 16 patients, while obstructive ventilatory disorder (OVD) was present in 32 patients, i.e. 66.6% of cases.

Table VI: Distribution of the population according to FEV1 value

FEV1 values(%)	*Number of patients*	*Frequency(%)*
>80	2	6,2
]60-80]	16	50
<60	14	43,7
Total	32	100

❖ Mimetic Beta2 reversibility test

Of the 32 patients with spirometry-objectified OVT, only 3 underwent further investigation using a beta-2 mimetic reversibility test. Significant reversibility was observed in all 3 cases. However, the mean value of the gain in FEV1 and FVC was not specified in the files.

❖ Non-specific bronchial provocation test with metacholine

Of the 10 patients with normal spirometry, ten underwent a non-specific bronchial provocation test with metacholine. This test was positive in 9 cases (Table VII).

Table VII: Results of the non-specific bronchial provocation test

Non-specific bronchial provocation test	*Number of patients*	*Frequency (%)*

Not realised	49	83
Realise	10	16,9
Positive	9	15,2
Negative	1	1,6

5. Confirmation of the occupational origin of asthma

5.1. Questioning data

5.1.1. Delay in onset of symptoms in relation to date of hire

The average time between the date of recruitment and the onset of respiratory problems was 9.33 ± 6.8 years. In 54.2% of cases, this time was between 5 and 15 years. In addition, 4 patients developed their first respiratory symptoms a few months after recruitment, while 6 others only became symptomatic after 20 years or more of exposure to the occupational risk (Figure 15).

In atopic subjects, respiratory symptoms appeared within an average of 6 years, with extremes ranging from a few months to 12 years. On the other hand, for non-atopic subjects, the average time was 10 years, with extremes ranging from a few months to 26 years.

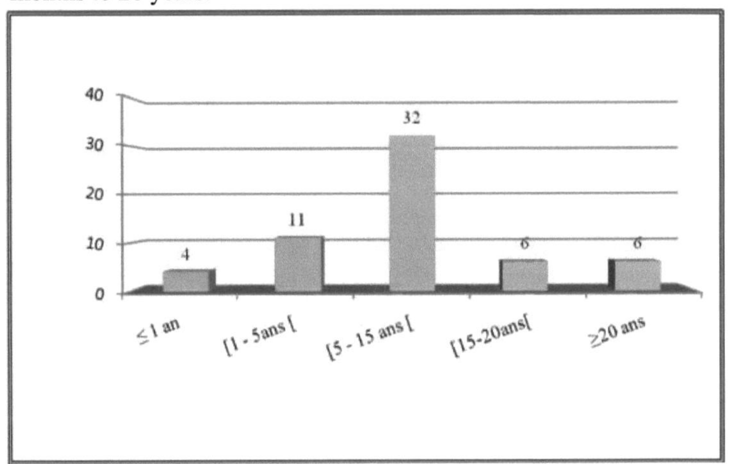

Figure 15: Distribution of the population according to the delay in onset of symptoms in relation to the date of recruitment

5.1.2. Age of symptoms

The average duration of symptoms before the first consultation was estimated at 4.42 ± 5 years, with extremes ranging from a few months to 24 years. Nearly two-thirds of patients (62%) consulted a specialist between one and five years after the onset of symptoms. Only 7 cases in the study population consulted within a few months of the onset of respiratory problems (Figure 16).

Number of patients

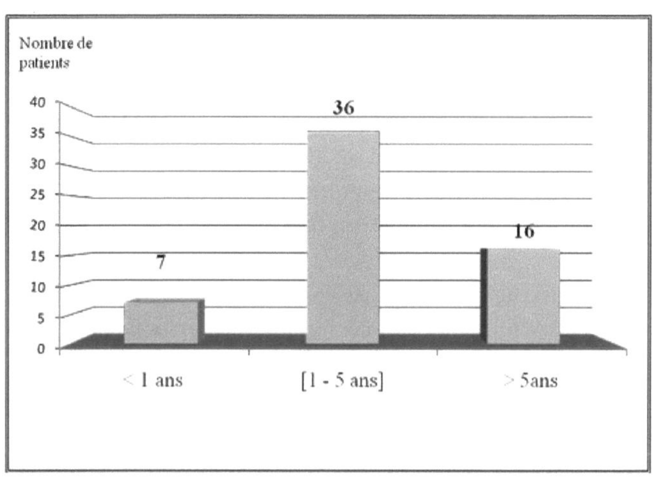

Figure 16: Breakdown of the population studied according to the consultation period

5.1.3. Rhythmic symptoms:

Symptomatology related to occupational exposure, with respiratory problems improving during weekly rest periods and/or annual leave and worsening during periods of activity, was reported by 25 patients (42.3%). On the other hand, this rhythmicity was not noted in 34 patients (57.6%).

5.2. Results of additional tests

5.2.1. Specific Ig E assay

Specific Ig E assays were performed in 14 patients (23.7%). Specific antibodies to one or more allergens were identified in 10 cases, i.e. 16.9% of the total population studied (Table VIII).

Table VIII: Results of the specific Ig E assay

Specific Ig E	*Number of patients*	*Frequency (%)*
Fact	14	23,7
Not done	45	76,2
Positive	10	16,9
Negative	4	6,7

Specific Ig E was tested for the following allergens:

- Plant dusts: 2 cases
- Methyl methacrylate: 1 case
- Cereals and flour: 3 cases
- Other agents responsible for allergic respiratory diseases: 2 cases
- Latex: 2 cases

- Isocyanates: 3 cases
- Nitro derivatives of phenol: 1 case study.

5.2.2. Staged spirometry

Thirteen patients underwent spirometry during exposure to the occupational risk, followed by spirometry after an interval of 7-10 days of allergen avoidance. An improvement in OVT without treatment was noted in 10 cases.

5.2.3. Specific bronchial provocation test

A specific bronchial provocation test was carried out in 4 patients in order to identify the causative agent of PA. In all 4 cases, the test was positive, enabling the diagnosis of PA to be made and the allergen (wood, flour, damp) to be specified. No notable incidents were attributed to these tests.

5.3. Professional survey

5.3.1. Workstation study

A workplace survey carried out by an investigator (engineer or safety technician) appointed by the CNAM was carried out for the entire population studied. Exposure to the suspected etiological agent was confirmed on questioning for 50 patients, i.e. 84.7% of reported cases (Table IX).

Table IX: Breakdown of the population according to job survey data

Job study	*Number of patients*	*Frequency (%)*
Carried out	59	100
Favourable	50	84,7
Not in favour	9	15,2

5.3.2. Aetiological agent involved

Flour and isocyanates are the two most common aetiological agents (17.8% each) (Figure 17).

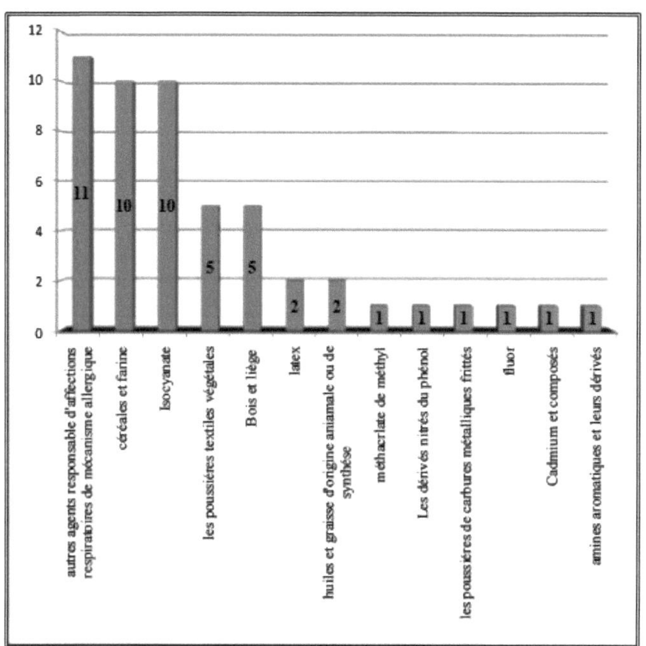

Figure 17: Breakdown of the study population by aetiological agent

90% of cases of PA caused by chemical agents, in particular isocyanates, come from the Sfax region, whereas 100% of cases recorded in Sidi Bouzid are caused by vegetable agents such as flour (Table X).

Table X: Breakdown of the study population by main regions and etiological agents

Region	Etiological agent	Number of cases
Sfax	Isocyanate	9
	Other chemical agents other than isocyante	5
	Flour	4
	Wood and cork	3
	Latex	1
Sidi Bouzid	Flour	3
	Plant textile dusts	4
	Plant dust	2
	Bois el liege	2

6. Legal and professional consequences

6.1. Declaration

The claim was made under various tables of occupational diseases (table XI), essentially the 3 following tables:

- Table 58: corresponding to other agents responsible for allergic respiratory diseases; 14 patients in our study were declared under this table.
- Table 56 on cereals and flour (14 other cases)
- Table 42 on Isocyanates (10 cases).

Table XI: Breakdown of the population by occupational disease table occupational diseases

Table No.	Painting title	Number of patients	Frequency(°%o)
10	Fluorine, hydrofluoric acid and its mineral salts	1	1,6
11	Cadmium and compounds	1	1,6
13	Sintered metal carbide dust	1	1,6
33	Aromatic amines and their derivatives	1	1,6
36	Nitro derivatives of phenols	1	1,6
39	Mineral and synthetic oils and fats	1	1,6
42	Isocyanates	10	16,9
44	Latex	1	1,6
53	Plant textile dusts	5	8,4
54	Wood and cork	5	8,4

56	Cereal flour	14	23,7
57	other plant dusts	4	6,7
58	other agents responsible for allergic respiratory diseases	14	23,7

6.2. Originating structure of the declaration

The breakdown of declared PA cases according to the structure of origin of the declaration is as follows (Table XII)

Hospital wards: 23 patients (38.9%);

Free-lance doctors: 19 patients (32.2%);

The occupational medicine groups (GMT) and the occupational medicine inspectorate (IMT): 15 patients (25.4%).

Table XII: Breakdown of the population studied by origin of declaration

Origin of declaration	Number of patients	Frequency (%)
Hospital services	23	38,9
Free-lance doctors	19	32,2
GMT / IMT	15	25,4
Occupational physicians	2	3,3

6.3. Recognition and rejection

Of the 59 HA cases reported, 38 cases were recognised, i.e. 64.4%, while 21 cases were rejected. The reasons for rejection were (Figure 18):

- Medical in 8 cases (13.5%);
- Administrative in 10 cases (16.9%);
- Medical and administrative in the 3 other cases (5%).

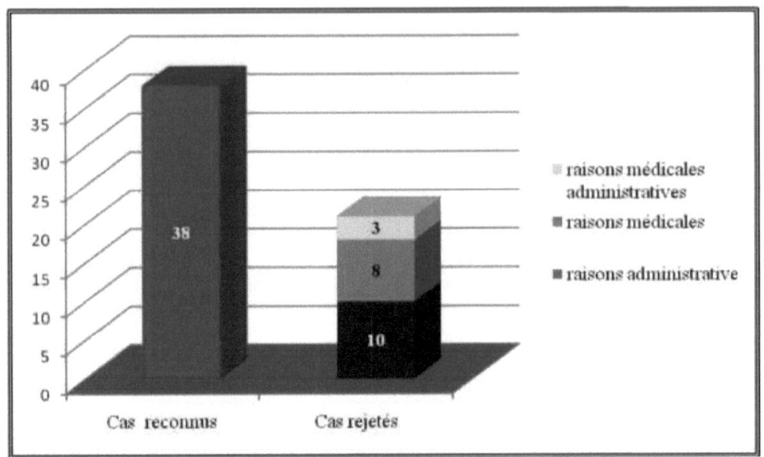

Figure 18: Distribution of the population studied according to recognition or rejection

The main medical and administrative reasons put forward to justify the rejection of certain declared cases:

- Medical reasons :

❖ No functional or physical signs in favour of asthma (3 cases),

❖ Normal EFR (3 cases) ;

❖ Positive skin test for non-occupational allergens (1 case);

❖ Industrial accident: massive exposure to the product (1 case).

- Administrative reasons

❖ Exceeding the deadline for taking charge.

1.4. Repair

As well as covering the cost of clinical and para-clinical investigations, the compensation procedure includes a permanent cash benefit awarded on the basis of the permanent partial disability (PPI) rate set by a specialised medical commission within the CNAM. The average rate of PPI awarded to patients receiving compensation was 24% (Figure 19).

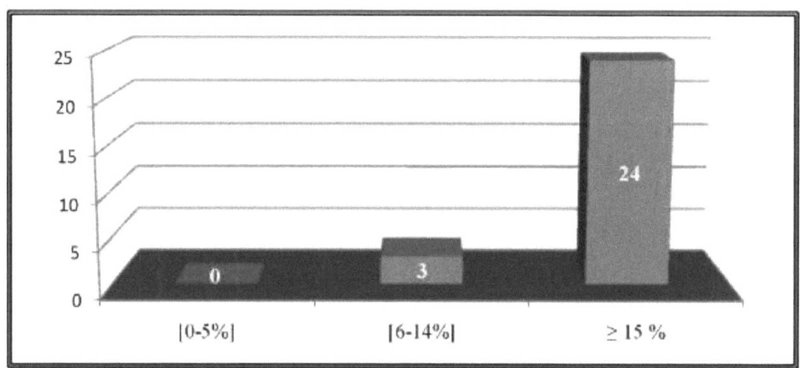

Figure 19 : Distribution of compensated cases according to the level of disability

1.5. Professional consequences

For recognised cases, the occupational outcome was as follows (Figure 20):
Retention of same workstation: 23 patients (60.5%).
Voluntary redundancies: 12 employees (31.5%).
Job transfer: 3 cases (7.8%).

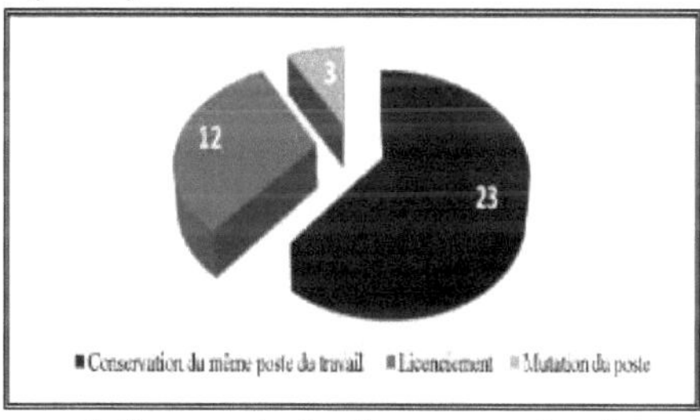

Figure 20: Breakdown of the population by occupational consequences

7. Treatment and development

7.1. Duration of follow-up

The average follow-up time was 2 ± 0.4 years, with extremes ranging from 4 months to 15 years.

7.2. Treatment

7.2.1. Eviction:

In our study, 12 out of 38 recognised cases opted for voluntary cessation of work and total allergen avoidance. The average duration of symptoms before eviction was 4.08 years.

7. 2.2. Medical treatment :

In our study, the health status of 20 patients required medical treatment in the case of gene for 5 patients and continuous background treatment combined with rescue treatment for the other 15. Despite total allergen avoidance, the health status of 10 patients who opted for a total work stoppage still required pharmacological treatment.

7.3. Evolution

Ten of the patients (16.9%) who stopped working reported a deterioration in their quality of life due to the persistent deterioration in their respiratory condition, which limited their daily activities, and a reduction in their income.

8. Analytical study

8.1. Predictors of PA severity

We used univariate analysis to identify factors predictive of asthma severity as judged by FEV1. In this study, the only factor significantly associated with disease severity in our cohort was the presence of a history of atopy ($p<0.01$) with a correlation index $r = 0.523$ (Table XIII).

Table XIII: Univariate analysis of PA severity according to variables of interest

Criteria	P
Gender	NS
Age	NS
Geographical origin	NS
Exposure time	NS
History of atopy	< 0.01
Nature of the causative agent	NS

8.2. PPI rate

There was a significant relationship between the PPI rate and FEV1 ($p= 0.06$) with a high correlation index ($r= -0.54$). However, there was no significant relationship with the other variables of interest (Table XIV).

Table XIV: Univariate analysis of the PPI rate as a function of the variables of interest

of interest

Criteria	P
Gender	NS
Age	NS
Geographical origin	NS
Duration of exposure to professional risk	NS
History of atopy	NS
Nature of the causative agent	NS

FEV1	0.06

4 DISCUSSION

1. Definition and limitations of our study

Several definitions have been proposed to characterise PA. They all emphasise the causal link between asthma and the work environment. Thus, PA has been defined as "an inflammation of the airways accompanied by variable bronchial obstruction and non-specific bronchial hyperreactivity induced by exposure to an agent present in the occupational environment" [6, 7, 8].

Two forms of PA are usually distinguished on the basis of clinical characteristics and the pathophysiological mechanisms involved [1, 8] (Table XV):

❖ Immunological (or "allergic") PA is characterised by bronchial hypersensitivity to an occupational substance, which appears after a latency period necessary for immuno-allergic sensitisation phenomena to take hold. This form of hypersensitivity can be caused by both high molecular weight (HPM) agents (e.g. proteins) and low molecular weight (FPM) agents (e.g. chemicals).

❖ Non-immunological PA is linked to acute toxicity induced by intense exposure to irritant substances and does not require a latency period. This "bronchial irritation syndrome" (BIS) has been described in the Anglo-Saxon literature as "reactive airways dysfunction syndrome" or "irritant induced asthma".

Table XV: Different types of occupational asthma [8].

	Occupational asthma	
	Immunological	*Non-immunological*
Mechanism	- Ig E dëpendant (HPM agents and certain FPM agents) - unknown (the majority of FPM agents)	Toxicity induced by single or multiple exposure to an irritant.
Clinical characteristics	- Latency period	- Acute onset - No latency period
Diagnosis	- Specific bronchial provocation test	- Time between exposure and onset of symptoms.

It should be noted that in our study we only included 1 immunological type of PA. SIB is often compensated as an accident at work (AT).

2. Descriptive epidemiology

2.1. Prevalence

2.1.1. Prevalence worldwide (Table XVI) :

PA is currently the most common work-related respiratory disease [5,9]. In fact, 10-15% of adult asthma is attributed to occupational activity [1,10], and this percentage is constantly rising [11].

However, prevalence surveys make it difficult to obtain a global approach because they are one-off studies of a limited number of specific occupational groups [12]. Some studies have made it possible to estimate the prevalence of PA in certain regions of the world:

❖ In Japan in 1980, 15% of all asthma was attributed to occupational exposure [13].

❖ In the USA in 1987, Blanc found a prevalence of 12,000 cases per million asthmatics [14].

❖ In 1999, a study carried out on 15637 people aged between 20 and 44 chosen at random from the general population of 26 regions in 12 industrialised countries (Belgium, Germany, Iceland, Ireland, Norway, Sweden, Italy, Spain, England, Australia, the United States and New Zealand) found an overall prevalence of PA of 5 to 10%. [15]

The PA prevalences studied depend on several factors, in particular the nature of the offending agent and, for the same agent, its concentration in the workplace and the handling conditions. Thus :

❖ Some studies report PA prevalences of up to 30% in animal workers, 5 to 25% in the case of exposure to isocyanates, and even up to 50% in the case of exposure to platinum salts or during the manufacture of laundry products (enzymes) [16].

❖ In 1999, Meyer et al. published data from the UK SWORD (surveillance of work related and occupational respiratory disease) register showing that rosin and other welding fluxes were responsible for 9% of PA cases recorded in the country during 1998. [17]

Table XVI: Prevalence of PA according to etiological agent (Based on the report by the Institut national de la sante et de la recherche research: INSERM)

Agents	***Profession/Industry***	***Prevalence (%)***	***Reference***
Laboratory animals	Laboratory workers	13	Venables et al. (1988)
Grain mite	Farmers	12	Cuthbert et al. (1984)
Papaine	Pharmaceutical industry	45	Baur et al. (1982)
Henne	hairstyle	17.4	Blainey et al. (1986)
Flour (wheat, rye, soya)	Bakers, millers	35	Musk et al. (1989)
Grain dust	Grain workers	40,47	Chan-Yeung et al (1980)

Latex	Glove manufacturers	6	Tarlo et al. (1990)

2.1.2. In Tunisia (Table XVII)

The retrospective nature of our work explains the underestimation of PA cases.

In our study, there was an almost even distribution of reported cases over the years, with a peak in 2004 (20.4%) and 2006 (16.9%).

In a study carried out in central Tunisia between 2000 and 2008 on 244 cases of PA, the mean annual frequency was 16.8% [18].

It is difficult to give an overall estimate of the prevalence of PA in Tunisia, since most of the studies carried out in our country are one-off studies with very different methodologies.

Table XVII: Examples of PA studies carried out in Tunisia [19].

Year	*Author*	*Sector - Agent*	*Workforce*	*Prevalence(%)*
1981	MRIZEK	Flour mill	126	1,6
1982	KLABI	Bakery	60	1,7
1982	KLABI	Joinery	400	0,5
1987	NOUAIGUI	Wood	197	5,7
1987	GHARBI	Textiles	797	7,8
1987	TURKI	Jute	285	2,1
1992	TAZEGHDENTI	Flour mill	389	0,8
1993	HAJEM	Tobacco	751	1,6
1997	ISST	Textiles	141	7,1
2001	TRABELSI	Hot plastics	129	3,9

In our study, plant origin was predominant (47.4% of cases compared with 32.2% for chemical origin).

2.2. Incidence

2.2.1. In the world

Numerous surveys have been carried out over the last 20 years to study the epidemiology of PA [10].

However, a marked lack of knowledge about this pathology [20] led to the creation of official systems for reporting occupational asthma in several industrialised countries [21]:

- In the United Kingdom: the Reporting of Injuries, Disease and Dangerous Occurrences Regulation (RIDDOR) and the Industrial Injuries Schemes [22].
- In Belgium, the Fonds des Maladies Professionnelles (FMP) [23].
- In Sweden: the Swedish Register of Reported Occupational Disease (SRROD) [24].
- In New Zealand: The Department of Labour Notifiable Occupational

Disease System registers notifications of new cases of occupational diseases [25].

❖ In Finland: a register was set up by the Finnish Institute of Occupational Health (FIOH) in 1964 [26].

In addition to these official systems, other voluntary reporting systems by doctors have been set up. Their aim is to provide a more comprehensive understanding of the incidence of HA.

❖ The SWORD system (Surveillance of Work Related and Occupational Respiratory Disease) was founded in 1989 in collaboration with the British Thoracic Society (BTS) and the Society of Occupational Medicine (SOM) [27].

❖ The SHIELD project was set up in 1989 in the West Midlands region of the United Kingdom [28].

❖ The SENSOR programme (Sentinel Event Notification System for Occupational Risks) was founded in 1987 in the United States [29].

❖ The PRIOR system was created in 1996 in the Piedmont region of Italy [30].

❖ In 1996, ONAP (1'observation nationale des asthmes professionnels) was set up in France by the Société de pneumologie de langue frangaise (SPLF) and the Société Frangaise de Medecine du Travail (SFMT) [31].

The PA incidence figures reported in various countries with voluntary surveillance systems are mostly between 20 and 40 cases/million workers (Table XVIII) [32].

Table XVIII: Estimated incidence of HA in various countries (voluntary declaration programme) [10].

Country	***Year***	***Incidence of ΓAP*** (per year and per million active workers)
Great Britain		
❖ SWORD	1989-92	22
	1992-93	37
❖ SHIELD	1990-97	41
United States(SENSOR) ❖ Michigan	1988-94	29
	1995	27
❖ California	1993-96	25
British Columbia	1991	92
Quebec	1992-93	42-79
	1997	26
France (ONAP)	1996-99	24
Italy (PRIOR)	1996-97	24
South Africa (SORDSA)	1997-99	17.,5

2.2.2. In Tunisia :

To date, there has been no national study of the overall incidence of HA in Tunisia.

According to our study, the average incidence of PA in southern Tunisia between 2002 and 2009 was 7.3 cases/year. Taking into account the size of the workforce in the Sfax region (100,000 workers), the incidence of this disease would be 40/100,000, which appears to be similar to the incidences reported in the literature, particularly in industrialised countries.

2.3. Age

The mean age of our population (42 ± 9.08 years) is close to that found in the literature (Table XIX):

Table XIX: Average age of subjects with PA according to the literature

Survey location	***Year***	***Average age in years***	***Reference***
Belgium	Between 2000 and 2002	39,3+/-11	[1]
Alsace	Between 2001 and 2002	36+/-11	[32]
Algeria	2004	- 34.5 (wood) - 36.2 (flour) - 45 (cotton) - 38.1 (leather)	[33]

2.4. Gender

Our study population was predominantly male (74.5%). This is in line with certain results found in the literature. For example, the ONAP found a clear male predominance (60.6%) in a population of 3,420 cases of PA. Similarly, in Belgium, out of 283 cases of PA reported between 2000 and 2002, two-thirds of patients (63.9%) were male [1].

In Alsace, on the other hand, E Popin et al found a slight predominance of women among all cases recorded by the ONAP between 2001 and 2002 [32].

2.5. Occupational category (Table XX)

In our study, blue-collar workers predominated (91.5%).

A pilot study (SENTASM) carried out in 2007-2008 in the Midi-Pyrenees region found that the prevalence of PA tended to be higher among unskilled workers than in other occupational categories (managers, higher intellectual professions, employees and skilled workers).

Table XX: Incidence rate (/100000) of HA according to social category professional [20]

Professional category	***Rates***
Teachers and others	18,7
Intermediate occupations in health and social work	16
Civil servants and public service employees	10,5
Commercial employees	10,4

Direct services to individuals	86
Skilled workers	162,9
Skilled craft workers	97,5
Skilled handling, storage and transport workers	30,2
Unskilled industrial workers	42,5
Unskilled craft workers	53,3

2.6. Sector of activity

Our population is spread across 16 different sectors of activity, led by the food industry (16 cases: 27.1%), followed by the wood industry (7 cases: 11.8%) and the metal construction industry (6 cases: 10.1%).

The study carried out at the Tunisian centre between 2000 and 2008 found that 62.1% of patients were employed in the garment sector and 12.8% in the spinning and textile sector, i.e. the % of workers reported for PA [19]. Similarly to our population, certain authors in New Zealand found a particularly high prevalence of PA in the agri-food industry sector [16, 34, 35].

This is also in line with the results reported by the ONAP (19.2% of PA declared between 1996 and 2001 came from the bakery and confectionery sectors) [20].

The literature review also shows that a significant percentage of PA has been noted in cleaning workers [15, 36, 37,38] (Table XXI).

Table XXI: Classification of the main occupations responsible for occupational asthma

occupational asthma, based on four monitoring programmes (from Kopferschmitt-Kubler et al. 1998) [39].

Profession	***NAPO (1996-97)***	***Finland (1990)***	***SHIELD (1989-91)***	***SWORD (1989-91)***
Baker	1	1	3	4
Professional of health	2	-	-	-
Car painter	3	2	1	1
Hairdresser	4	-	-	-
Woodworking professions	5	-	4	6
Textile industry	6	-	-	-
Farmer	-	3	-	-
Welder	-	4	6	5
Plastics industry	-	-	2	2
Chemical treatment	-	-	5	3

3. Pathophysiology

3.1. Predisposing (or risk) factors

3.1.1. Individual risk factors

3.1.1.1. Atopy

In our study, there was only one case of familial atopy, while personal antecedents of atopy were found in 13 patients (22%).

Atopy is defined as a personal or familial tendency to produce specific Ig E in response to low doses of allergens and to develop typical clinical manifestations such as asthma, rhinitis, conjunctivitis or eczema [40].

Several studies have shown that the existence of an atopic background increases the risk of developing PA to high molecular weight occupational agents [41, 42,43]. However, atopy does not appear to favour the development of allergic asthma to HMW agents [44,45].

However, the positive predictive value of atopy is fairly low, and there does not seem to be any ethical justification for recommending the systematic exclusion of atopic subjects from exposed occupations [46].

In a series of 25 employees with PA, 22 subjects (88%) had rhinitis and asthma as antecedents. For 17 of them, rhinitis symptoms preceded respiratory symptoms [47].

3.1.1.2. Smoking

Smoking intoxication was not studied in our population, given the retrospective nature of this study.

Although its role in the genesis of PA has not been clearly established [48,49], several authors have considered smoking to be a risk factor for sensitisation to MPF agents acting by an Ig E-dependent mechanism, thus favouring the onset of asthma (this is the case for platinum salts and anhydride compounds) [50,51].

On the other hand, smoking does not appear to be a factor favouring asthma to MPF agents acting by an independent Ig E mechanism: non-smokers would even be more susceptible than smokers to asthma to red cedar or isocyanates [52].

In 2008, S. Monier et al showed that smoking was not a cofactor in wood dust asthma [53].

The mechanism by which cigarette smoking may promote certain types of asthma is not known, but is thought to be linked on the one hand to the increased synthesis of immunoglobulin E in smokers in relation to HPM agents, and on the other hand to the increased permeability of the bronchial mucosa to potential allergens due to the irritative effect of tobacco on the bronchial mucosa [50,54].

Venables et al found a synergistic interaction between atopy and smoking in animal laboratory workers [55] and in those exposed to tetrachlorophthalic

anhydride [51] .
Some studies have shown that smoking rather than atopy is the most important factor in the development of PA in workers in animal laboratories and platinum refineries [55,56].

3.1.1.3. Non-specific bronchial hyperreactivity:

This is an essential, but not specific, characteristic of asthmatics [57].
The available data do not allow us to state definitively that the existence of asthma and/or non-specific bronchial hyperreactivity increases the risk of developing PA [13].
Furthermore, the extent to which HRBNS is a result of exposure or is a predisposing factor for PA remains a controversial issue. Chan-Yeung and Malo suggest that HRBNS is the result of exposure to occupational aerocontaminants and not a predisposing factor in the development of the disease [58]. These two authors demonstrated in a longitudinal study that PA induced by red cedar dust occurred in workers who did not have HRBNS before the onset of work-related asthmatic symptoms [59].
However, a recent study of a cohort of apprentices exposed to laboratory animals showed that the onset of PA was significantly more frequent in subjects with HRBNS prior to exposure to the offending allergens [60].

3.1.1.4. HLA status (Table XXII)

A relationship between PA caused by MPF agents (e.g. isocyanates) and certain HLA class II antigens involved in the presentation of the antigen to immune cells has been described by some authors [61,62].
Workers carrying the DQei-0503 allele in their HLA class II genetic typing or DQei -0201/0301 combinations would be more likely to develop asthma attributable to isocyanates.

Table XXII: *Genetic factors involved in PA [10].*

Professional agent	Number of subjects	Gene	Association (RR)	Reference
Isocyanate	28 TPS +	❖ HLA DQB1 *0503 ❖ HLA DQB1*0201/*0301 ❖ HLA DQB1 *0501 ❖ HLA DQA1*0101 and or *0102	9 ,8 9,5 0,1 0,1	[61]
Isocyanate	30 + GST	❖ HLA DQB1 *0503 ❖ HLA DQB1 *0501	2,9 0,1	[63]
Isocyanate	67 TPS+	❖ HLA DQB1*0503 ❖ HLA DQA1*0104 ❖ HLA DQB1*0501 ❖ HLA DQA1*0101	ND ND ND ND	[64]
Isocyanate	55 (7 TPS +)	* HLA DRB1/DQB1/DQA1	Absent	[65]
Isocyanate	10 GST / PED+ (IN FRENCH)	* HLA- DR/DQ	Absent	[66]
Isocyanate	142 (106 TPS+)	❖ HLA - A, B, C ❖ TNF a-308 polymorphism	Absent Absent	[67]
Acid anhydride	30 I g E +	* HLA- DR3	6	[68]
Acid anhydride	52 I g E +	❖ HLA - DQ 5	4,3	[69]

		❖ HLA- DQB1*0501 ❖ HLA- DR1	3 3	
Turntable	44 CT +.	❖ HLA- DR3 ❖ HLA- DR6	2,3 0,4	[70]
Latex	189 Ig E +	❖ HLA- DQB1*0302 ❖ HLA- DRB1*04	ND ND	[71]
Rat (urinary allergen)	109 Ig E / TC	❖ HLA- DR7 ❖ HLA- DR3	1,8 0,5	[72]
Isocyanate	109 TPS/DEP+	❖ GSTM1 nil ❖ GSTM1 null + GSTM3AA	1,8 ND	[73]
Isocyanate	109 TPS/DEP+	❖ NAT1 ❖ GSTM1 null + NAT1 ❖ GSTM1 null + NAT2	2,5 4,5 3,1	[74]
Isocyanate	56 TPS +	❖ GSTMP1	0,2	[75]

TPS+ : AP demonstrated by a positive specific bronchial provocation test; DEP + : AP demonstrated by recording peak expiratory flow; TC + positive skin test for the allergen; Ig E + presence of immunoglobulin specific for the causative agent; GSTM glutathione S transferase; NAT : n- acetyl transferase.

Other authors have reported an association between isocyanate-induced PA and certain genotypes of glutathione S-transferase and N-acetyl transferase, which play a vital role in protecting cells against oxidative damage [73].

On the whole, these associations are fairly weak, and do not currently allow the use of genetic tests to be envisaged for the identification of workers at risk of developing PA [10].

3.2. Environmental factors in the workplace

Overall, epidemiological studies show that the intensity of exposure to sensitising agents is the main risk factor on which PA prevention efforts should therefore focus.

There is a dose-response relationship between the intensity of exposure and the prevalence of immunological sensitisation to various occupational agents such as laboratory animals [76], cereal meal [77] and latex [41].

Although it is currently impossible to assert the existence of an exposure threshold below which Ig E sensitisation and AP do not occur [10], the available data suggest that the risk is minimal when exposure levels are below 0,5 mg/m3 for flour dust, 0.2 Lig/m3 for wheat allergens [77], 0.25 ng/m3 for l'a-amylase [78], 0.7 Lig/m3 for rat urine allergens [79] and 0.6 ng/m3 for natural latex allergens [80].

The effect of environmental factors remains difficult to assess because of the "healthy worker effect", defined as the tendency of workers to leave their jobs because of the severity of their symptoms [81].

3.3. Etiological factors:

The agents most implicated in the generation of PA identified during our study are isocyanates and flour. Their distribution differs from one town to another according to the predominant economic sector. Thus, plant origin is characteristic of the region of Sidi Bouzid, where agricultural activity predominates, whereas chemical origin predominates in the region of Sfax, which is an industrial town.

A review of the literature shows that there are a large number of agents providing PA: J.L MALO [42] estimates that there are more than 250 and J.Ameille [10] nearly 300. Their distribution differs from country to country according to the predominant economic sectors.

They can be subdivided according to their size into high- and low-molecular agents (Table XXIII), according to the immunological mechanism they induce into Ig E-dependent and other Ig E-independent agents, and according to the latency period required for clinical manifestations to appear into factors causing asthma with or without a latency period (Table XXIV) [42].

Table XXIII: Characteristics of high and low molecular weight agents causing PA [42].

Agent characteristics	High molecular weight	Low molecular weight
Agent size	>5 KD	< 5 KD
Immunological mechanism	Ig E	Generally unknown
Latency period	Longer	Shorter

In France, the results are similar to our study and the main causes of PA are flour, isocyanates, latex and persulphates [3].

Table XXIV: Breakdown of etiological factors in agents of PMH and PMF

HPM agents	**FPM agents**
❖ Cereals ❖ Phaneres and excrement of animals ❖ Enzymes ❖ Latex ❖ Food and miscellaneous ❖ Mould	❖ Wood ❖ Isocyanates ❖ Metals ❖ Resins, paint, glue ❖ Biocide ❖ Welding ❖ Chloramine T ❖ Dyes, colorants ❖ Persulphates ❖ Formaldehydes, glutaraldehydes ❖ Methacrylates ❖ Medicines ❖ Amine ❖ Acid anhydride

❖ .2.1. HPM substances

3.2.1.1.. Enzymes

Enzymes are used in a wide range of industries. If they are handled in pulverulent or aerosolised form, they constitute an occupational risk of respiratory sensitisation and therefore of the onset of PA.

Alpha amylase is one of the enzymes most classically implicated in baker's asthma [82].

The other PA-producing enzymes are summarised in Table XXV.

Table XXV: Enzymes responsible for AP [3,83]

(Non-exhaustive list)

Detergents industry	❖ Protease (exp alpha amylase) ❖ Subtilisin ❖ Lipase ❖ Cellulase
Enzyme production and biotechnology research	❖ Cellulase ❖ Xylanase
Pharmaceutical industry	❖ Trypsin ❖ Chymotrypsin ❖ Brombline ❖ Cellulase ❖ Pepsin
Bakery	❖ Alpha amylase ❖ Gluco amylase ❖ Xylanase, ❖ cellulase
Other areas of the food industry	❖ Alpha amylase ❖ Xylanase, ❖ Cellulase ❖ Papain

3.2.1.2. Allergens from the food industry

Food industry workers are exposed to a considerable number of allergens responsible for PA, such as products of marine origin [84] and egg proteins [85]. Respiratory reactions result from aerosols generated during the cleaning, preparation, cooking or drying of food [3].

In our study, the main food-borne agent incriminated was flour (16.9% of cases).

3.2.1.3. Allergens in agriculture

The prevalence of asthma in the agricultural environment is between 3 and 7.7% [86].

Allergens can come from :

❖ Vegetable: pollen, moulds, cereals, oilseeds and protein crops, textile fibres, various plants, wood, etc.

- ❖ Animal: mammalian allergens (horses, cattle, pigs...), poultry and bird allergens, arthropod allergens, insect allergens.
- ❖ Chemical: insecticides, herbicides, fungicides, antibiotics, anti-parasitics.

❖ .2.2. FPM substances

Isocyanates, chemical compounds frequently used in the manufacture of polyurethanes, are the leading cause of PA to chemical agents [3].

According to ONAP data in France, this substance, along with flour, latex and persulphate aldehydes, accounts for 50% of PA cases [10].

In our study, isocyanates were the leading cause of chemical PA (16.9% of all cases).

Several industrial activities involve the use of isocyanates:

- ❖ Gluing wood
- ❖ Varnishing furniture
- ❖ Bonding leather and ceramics
- ❖ Electrical and thermal insulation, sealing joints
- ❖ Automotive industry (body paint, upholstery, seats, car cushions, etc.)
- ❖ Manufacture and use of anti-corrosion paints
- ❖ Protective foams for packaging
- ❖ Manufacture of sailboards and pleasure boats.

In our study, isocyanates are used mainly in the metal construction, joinery and wood and foam industries.

3.4. Pathogenic mechanisms (Figure 21)

Depending on the nature of the causative agent, the pathogenic mechanism involved is either immunological (Ig E-dependent or -independent) or non-immunological.

3.4.1. Immunological (or allergic) mechanism

This mechanism is characterised by a latency period required for the onset of immuno-allergic sensitisation [8].

3.4.1.1. Immunological mechanism, Ig E dependent

The majority of HPM agents (> 5000 daltons) induce AP through the production of specific antibodies (specific Ig E) directed against the agent in question. Some MPF agents (e.g. platinum salts, trimellitic anhydride and other acid anhydrides) act by a similar mechanism, leading in turn to the synthesis of specific Ig E antibodies. Due to their small size, these substances are unable to act as allergens on their own and must combine with a carrier protein to express themselves as haptenes [87].

The production of an immune response involves a series of cascading reactions [88] :

❖ Activation of T lymphocytes: the TCR (T cell receptor) recognises the antigenic peptide attached to an MHC (major histocompatibility complex) class I or II molecule on the surface of cells presenting the "CPA" antigen (macrophages, dendritic cells and B lymphocytes).

❖ The CPA facilitates this process of recognition and therefore activation of the T lymphocytes (LT) by producing IL1, which stimulates the LT.

❖ Active T lymphocytes secrete lymphokines that attract and activate the growth and differentiation of other leukocytes (mast cells, eosinophils, macrophages, B lymphocytes).

* TH1 secretes IL-2 and interferon-Y (IFN-Y)
* TH2 secretes IL-4 and IL-5.
* TH1 and TH2 secret IL3 and GM-CSF.

❖ Active mast cells release 2 types of mediators

* Preformed mediators (histamine; leukotrienes C4, D4, and E4; and prostaglandin D2) then cause early bronchoconstriction.
* Cytokines and adhesion molecules involved in the delayed inflammatory reaction after allergen exposure has been stopped [89].

❖ Activation of eosinophils and B lymphocytes whose action is similar to that produced during allergic asthma [16]. (eosinophils: secretion of cytotoxic proteins and interleukins, B lymphocytes: (differentiated into plasma cells) production of Ig E-specific antibodies).

❖ Produced in large quantities, specific Ig E binds to high-affinity receptors (Fc) on the surface of mast cells and basophils and to low-affinity receptors on the surface of eosinophils, macrophages, platelets and epithelial cells, stimulating the production of inflammatory mediators.

3.3.I.2 Immunological mechanism, Ig E independent :

Most MPF agents, such as isocyanates, red cedar and acrylates, cause an AP whose clinical characteristics are similar to Ig E-dependent immunological AP but which does not systematically induce the production of specific Ig E [8,90].

Specific Ig E may be found in some patients. When these immunoglobulins are present, they are probably only markers of exposure, and not the cause of the disease [13,87].

The inflammatory process involved is similar to that involved in Ig E-dependent AP, the only difference being that T lymphocytes release cytokines capable of activating and recruiting other inflammatory cells, thus acting as effector cells via pathways different from those of Ig E production [87].

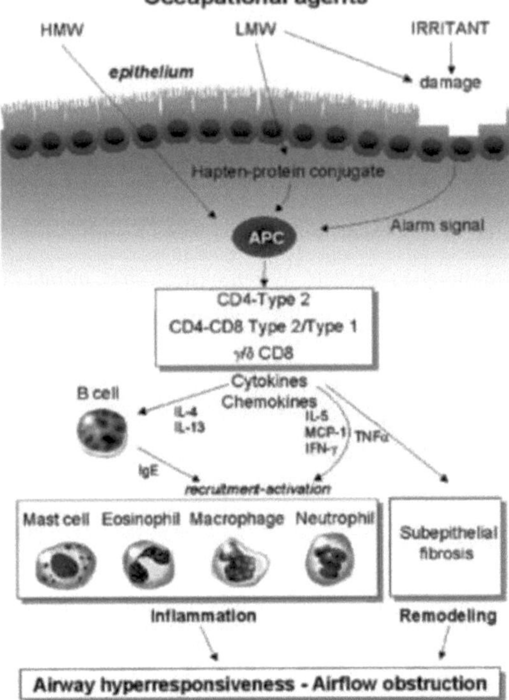

Figure 21: Schematisation of possible pathophysiological mechanisms of PA [87].

3.3.2. Non-immunological (or non-allergic) mechanism

Non-immunological AP is characterised by the absence of a latency period, with acute onset of symptoms following a single or multiple exposure to high doses of the allergen [8].

The pathophysiological mechanism of this type of asthma is not fully understood [87]. Some authors explain it by the toxic effect of inhaled irritants on the mucous membrane of the airways. This effect results in the loss of relaxation factors in the bronchial epithelium and the exposure of nerve endings, which triggers a neurogenic inflammatory process. In addition, this aggression leads to the release of inflammatory mediators, with possible activation of the non-cholinergic non-adrenergic system (NANC) and release of neurokinins.

4. Diagnosis

There are two stages in diagnosing 1 AP:

❖ Making a positive diagnosis of asthma

❖ Demonstrate its occupational origin.

4.1. Affirming asthma

4.1.1. Clinical study

4.1.1.1. Asthma attacks [91,92,93].

In its typical form, an asthma attack develops rapidly, often preceded by prodromal symptoms (respiratory signs: rhinorrhea, sneezing, dry cough, nasal pruritus; behavioural problems: irritability, anxiety; ocular signs: lacrimation, conjunctivitis, ocular pruritus, ocular ringing, etc.).

Clinical signs include dyspnoea, cough, chest tightness and sibilance on auscultation. It subsides after a few minutes to several hours, more rapidly after inhalation of a в2 mimetic. It is followed by a phase of productive cough, known as "Laennec sputum".

Reversibility and variability are two important elements to look for.

The absence of an attack on the day of the examination and/or sibilant rales on lung auscultation does not rule out the diagnosis.

In our study, 74.5% of patients reported wheezing.

4.1.1.2. Asthma with continuous dyspnea:

This is an advanced form of severe asthma in adults, combining permanent dyspnoea with sibilants and exacerbations, which are often severe. There is fixed bronchial obstruction on EFR [91].

4.1.2. Paraclinical diagnosis

4.1.2.1. Confirmation of reversible bronchial obstruction

❖ Spirometry and beta 2 mimetic test

Although non-specific, the demonstration of reversible bronchial obstruction is a fundamental element in the diagnosis of bronchial asthma. Spirometry should therefore be part of the evaluation and follow-up of any patient suspected of having asthma (Figure 23) [91]. The ERS (European Respiratory Society) criteria for obstruction are an FEV1/FVC ratio (Tiffeneau ratio) of less than 88% of theoretical for men and less than 89% of theoretical for women [16]. Reversibility of obstruction is defined by an increase in FEV1 of at least 12% (or 200 ml in absolute value) compared with baseline values, after inhalation of a fast-acting в2 mimetic. However, the absence of a response does not exclude the diagnosis and the test can then be repeated after a 15-day course of oral glucocorticoids (prednisone 0.5 mg/kg/d) [94].

Outside an attack, respiratory function may be normal, which again does not exclude the diagnosis of asthma, the characteristic feature of which is variability. [91]

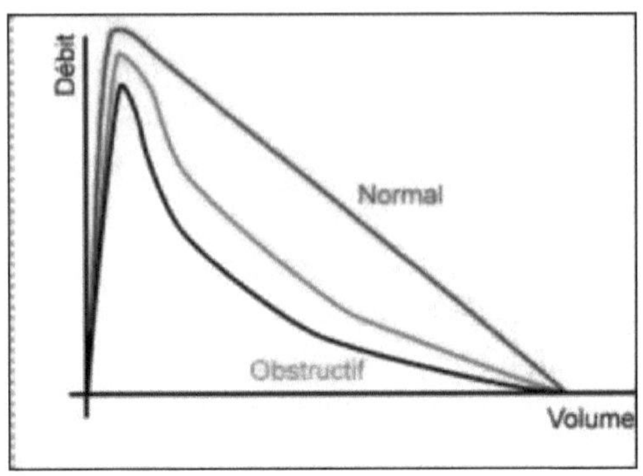

Figure 22: appearance of the spirometry curve in normal conditions and in the case of OVT

Spirometry performed on 48 patients in our population showed OVT in 66.6% of cases. Thirteen of these patients with a TVO had a reversibility test with beta 2 mimetic, which showed a reversible TVO in all cases.

Our results are similar to those found in a study of all PA cases in Alsace in 2001-2002: 33% of reported cases underwent spirometry, which revealed OVT in 87% of cases [32].

Furthermore, in a study carried out at the Tunisian centre on all PA cases recorded between 2000 and 2008, 60.3% of all cases who underwent spirometry had a TVO [18].

❖ State-of-the-art debimetry :

When spirometry is normal, the diagnosis of asthma can be aided by looking for daytime variability in peak expiratory flow (PEF) [91].

❖ Search for non-specific bronchial hyperreactivity (NSAH) :

Non-specific bronchial hyperresponsiveness is defined as excessive obstruction of the bronchi in response to various stimuli that produce little or no response in normal individuals. It is an essential, but non-specific, feature of asthma [57].

Many patients presenting with a clinical history suggestive of asthma may, however, present without sibilance on clinical examination and have a normal baseline EFR. In these cases, the demonstration of a methacholine HRBNS is an additional diagnostic argument. This test makes it possible to detect hyper-reactive cases among dyspnoeic subjects and chronic coughers with a normal spirometric and clinical examination.

In our study, HRBNS was investigated by a non-specific metacholine challenge test in 10 patients with normal baseline spirometry. This test was positive in 9 of them.

4.1.2.2. Confirmation of an allergic (or atopic) background

❖ Biological characteristics of allergy :
In our study, hyper eosinophilia was found in 3 patients and an increase in total Ig E was found in 11 patients (18.6%).

❖ Standard skin tests
Skin tests (CT) have always played an important role in allergology.
Skin tests (prick test) with an immediate reading at fifteen minutes have good specificity but lower sensitivity than intradermal tests [96].
During the course of our study, 27 patients benefited from a prick test, which proved positive in 18 patients (66.6% of cases).

❖ ORAL examination
Epidemiological studies have shown that asthma and rhinitis are very often associated in atopic patients [97].
In the case of allergic bronchial asthma, an ENT examination (including a rhinoscopic examination and possibly a sinus CT scan) should be carried out to look for rhinitis and/or nasal polyposis [98,99].

4.2. Asserting the occupational origin of asthma

4.2.1. Questioning

In an update published in 2006, G Pauli set out the main useful questions to ask [5]:

❖ Questions about symptomatology:
* Asthma (stagc, activity, severity...)
* Asthma equivalents and atypical manifestations (spasmodic cough, dyspnoea...)
* Associated symptoms (rhinoconjunctivitis, urticaria, etc.)
* Clinical signs of HRBNS.

❖ Questions about the chronology of symptoms
* Delay between symptoms and exposure
* Onset of symptoms in relation to work.
* Stop and restart test
* Improvement during holidays
* Atopy, smoking, pre-existing asthma, previous accidental exposure.

According to the American College of Chest Physicians (ACCP), 5 questions are useful in the initial diagnostic approach to clarify whether the symptoms presented by the employee are really due to occupational exposure: [100] 1) Were there any changes in work procedures during the period preceding the onset of your symptoms?
2) Were there any unusual occupational exposures in the last 24 hours (an affirmative answer to this question points to "bronchial irritation syndrome")?

3) Do asthma symptoms differ during periods of absence from work (holidays and bank holidays)?
4) Do the symptoms of allergic rhinitis and conjunctivitis worsen during labour? (a positive response suggests specific sensitisation during labour).
5) Are there other workers with the same symptoms?
A negative response to all of these questions is associated with a low probability of PA. A positive answer or more is not sufficient for diagnosis, but should lead to more specialised investigations.
The sensitivity of questioning for the diagnosis of PA appears to be good (80 to 93%) but its specificity is generally less than 50% (Table XXVI) [101].
The limitations of questioning are linked to a number of factors [9] :

❖ Lack of objective assessment of symptoms (the patient may exaggerate or, on the contrary, minimise complaints, atypical symptoms: cough preceding asthma not taken into account).

❖ Atypical chronology

❖ Difficulty in linking symptoms to a precise etiological agent in the case of intermittent exposure.

Furthermore, the positive predictive value of a suggestive clinical history is mediocre. In fact, the reduction in symptoms observed during periods of occupational avoidance may also be observed in patients with non-occupational asthma. Similarly, the symptoms of these asthmatics may be triggered or aggravated by exposure to occupational exposure.
irritants in the workplace [101]. Thus, questioning is more useful in excluding than in confirming the diagnosis of PA.
Some important concepts need to be clarified in the analysis
1) Delay in the onset of symptoms in relation to the date of recruitment: "latency period
In our study, the mean time to onset of symptoms was 9.33+/- 6.81 years (111.96+/-81.72). Four patients experienced their first symptoms immediately after recruitment (a few weeks to a few months), which could be due to bronchial irritation syndrome or to previous exposure that was unrecognised or neglected.
In PA, the time between the onset of exposure and the first symptoms varies from a few weeks to several years [6]. This delay favours the diagnosis of de novo asthma acquired in the workplace [16].
O Vandenplas et al. found in a study of all cases reported between 2000 and 2002 in Belgium a latency period of 92+/- 108 months [1], which is close to our results.

2) Consultation deadline

The average time between onset of clinical symptoms and first consultation for our population was 4.42+/- 5.02 years (53.04+/- 60.23 months), which is very similar to the results found by O Vandenplas et al. in a study of all reported cases of PA between 2000 and 2002 in Belgium (consultation time in months 44+/- 72 months) [1].

3) Rhythmicity of symptoms

The notion that symptoms improve during periods of absence from work (leave, holidays) and reappear when work is resumed is a fundamental element to be clarified during the initial investigation of a PA [100].

A worsening or onset of asthma symptoms in the workplace (sick leave tests, improvement during leave) is a good argument in favour of the occupational origin of asthma [16].

In our study, 25 patients (42.3%) had symptoms associated with occupational exposure. However, this rhythmicity tends to disappear with the age of the asthma, with dyspnea gradually overtaking periods of rest, with improvement only occurring after increasingly prolonged periods of rest [10].

In our study, PA was diagnosed in 20 of the 25 patients who presented with a clinical history suggestive of PA (functional respiratory symptoms that worsen during periods of work and disappear or improve after eviction). However, 18 of the 36 patients whose clinical history was not suggestive of PA actually had the disease. In our study, the sensitivity of the history was 52.6% and the specificity 76.1%.

Table XXVI: Validity of the clinical history in the diagnosis of PA [101].

Agent	*Number of subjects*	*Number of subjects with a clinical history suggestive of PA*	*Sensitivity (%)*	*Specificity (%)*
Miscellaneous	162	104	87	22
Red cedar	23	-	93	45
Miscellaneous	204	-	80	55
Latex	45	-	87	14
Latex	30	30	89	50

Table XXVII: Validity of the clinical history in the diagnosis of PA in our series

Agent	*Number of subjects*	*Number of subjects with a clinical history suggestive of PA*	*Sensitivity*	*Specificity % (%)*
Various	59	25	52,6	76,1

4) Functional symptoms

* Thoracic symptoms

In our study, the main complaint reported by patients was wheezing (44 patients;

74.5%), while 13 patients (22%) had a dry cough. Almost half the population (25 patients, 42.3%) had multiple symptoms (dyspnea and/or cough associated with extra-thoracic atopic manifestations).

Our results corroborate those of the literature. According to which the main complaints are either typical asthma symptoms (wheezing) or asthma equivalents (spasmodic cough, chest tightness, clinical signs of bronchial hyperreactivity such as coughing on smoking, strong odours, etc.) [16,89].

J. Kongerud et al. have shown that the sensitivity and specificity of a question relating to the presence or absence of dyspnea in the workplace are good (83%, 79% respectively); the same is true for a question relating to the existence or absence of a cough (sensitivity 73%; specificity 67%).

* Associated atopic symptoms:

In our study population, 22 patients (37.2%) developed extra-thoracic atopic manifestations after recruitment (allergic rhinitis: 19 patients; rhinoconjunctivitis: 1 patient and allergic eczema: 3 patients).

The association of extra- thoracic allergic manifestations (mainly allergic rhinitis but also ocular and cutaneous manifestations) with PA is a phenomenon frequently described in the literature [102]. These atopic manifestations were attested by the presence of specific Ig E or by the positivity of a specific skin test [2].

According to N Rosenberg, in a study of occupational respiratory allergies caused by wood dust, the rate of PA associated with rhinitis was 55-70% [103]. Surber in 1977 noted the very high frequency of rhino-sinus manifestations (56%) among 96 Swiss carpenters and cabinet makers, 2.1% of whom suffered from PA [104].

J-L. Malo et al. showed that the prevalence of rhinoconjunctivitis was greater with PA due to HPM agents than with PA due to FPM agents [105].

4.2.2. Professional survey

For all the cases of PA studied in our series, a workplace investigation was carried out by a qualified CNAM agent. This was conclusive for 50 cases and ruled out suspected exposure for 9 patients. The data from this investigation for our patients was limited to determining whether or not there had been exposure to the etiological agent listed on the CMI or the workplace declaration.

This investigation is an essential step in the diagnosis of PA [13]. It must not only confirm whether or not the patient is exposed to the incriminating etiological agent in the workplace, but also :

❖ List all the products handled in the workstation and in neighbouring workstations.

❖ Identify how these products are used and the conditions under which they are handled (hot or cold, enclosed environment, etc.)

❖ Specify whether or not protective equipment is used

❖ If necessary, take samples of the products handled (which can be used as allergens for prick tests) and determine their atmospheric concentrations.

❖ Obtain the safety data sheet for the products used, detailing their chemical composition, impact on health, safety instructions for use, metabolism and toxicological data.

4.2.3. Paraclinical diagnosis

4.2.3.1. Functional respiratory investigations (FRI)

* Sequential measurement of PEF and stepped spirometry:

Variations in spirometric recording and PEF induced by occupational exposure are a valuable aid in attesting the occupational nature of asthma [32,47].

Recording PEF at work and outside work, and measuring FEV1 at the beginning and end of a working day to detect fluctuations in the values recorded, are often presented as simple and inexpensive methods for investigating PA (Table XXVIII) [101].

Some authors have proposed twice-daily measurement of PEF [5], while others recommend four measurements per day, recording symptoms and treatments at the same time [106]. A study by J. Malo et al. showed that the specificity and sensitivity of four measurements of PEF during a working day is similar to those of measuring PEF every 2 hours [107]. At each measurement, the patient records his PEF 3 times in succession and retains the best value of the 3 [95].

According to current recommendations, iterative measurement of PEF should be performed over a minimum period of 4 weeks, including one week off work [47]. During this period, the patient should not receive any treatment apart from short-acting Beta-2 mimetics on demand. However, if a treatment was initiated before the monitoring period, it should not be modified during the measurement period. It is therefore advisable to replace long-acting B2-mimetics with short-acting B2-mimetics [6].

It has been shown that extending the period of iterative measurement of PEF (4 weeks versus 2 weeks) improves its sensitivity and specificity [108].

Intraday variability of more than 20 or 25% strongly suggests a diagnosis of PA [13].

However, sequential measurement of PEF has certain disadvantages: [6, 9,13]

❖ intermittent exposure to the professional agent can be a factor in error.

❖ DEP monitoring cannot formally identify the agent responsible in the event of simultaneous exposure to several potential etiological agents.

❖ recording of PEF in the workplace should not be carried out if there is a history of severe asthmatic reaction in the workplace.

❖ make sure that the work DEP measurement is carried out at the patient's previous workstation.

❖ Biases due to recording by the patient him/herself.

❖ It cannot be used for illiterate people.

In our series, sequential recording of PEF was not performed. Longitudinal spirometry (stepped) was performed for 13 patients according to the following protocol:

- Spirometry recording during the period of occupational exposure (the patient works under the usual conditions)
- A second recording is made after a period of absence from work ranging from one week to two weeks.

> The exploration was considered positive if

- The initial recording is normal and the second documents a TVO.
- A variation in FEV1 > 12% between the 2 recordings.

> The sensitivity and specificity of this investigation in our study were good (83.3% and 100% respectively).

A review of the literature shows that sequential FEV1 measurement has good sensitivity and specificity for the diagnosis of PA, which supports our results.

Table XXVIII: Validity of PEF monitoring in the diagnosis of PA [101].

Agent	*Number of subjects*	*SensibiUte(°%)*	*Specificity(%)*
Red cedar	23	86	89
Miscellaneous	50	93	70
Red cedar	25	87	90
Various	61	81	74
Various	74	73	78
Various	20	73	100
Various	49	35	65

Table XXIX: Validity of PEF monitoring in the diagnosis of PA in our study

Agent	*Number of subjects*	*SensibiUte(°%)*	*Specificity(%)*
Miscellaneous	59	83,3	100

* Non-specific bronchial hyperresponsiveness (NSBRH):

In addition to its value in contributing to the positive diagnosis of asthma, the demonstration of a change in HRBNS following exposure to incriminating occupational agents can attest to the link between asthma and work.

Measurement of HRBNS as a function of work activity is especially recommended in uncooperative patients in order to perform a PEF diary [6]. HRBNS may decrease or even disappear after eviction of the causal agent and reappear or increase again after re-exposure [101].
However, the absence of HRBNS makes it possible to exclude, with virtual certainty, the diagnosis of PA if the test was performed in the immediate aftermath of exposure to the offending substance [109]. However, HRBNS may be missing, and the proportion of cases of isocyanate-induced PA with negative tests for cholinergic mediators varies, depending on the study, from 10 to 20% [6].
It seems unfortunate that the HRBNS in a number of our patients was only measured once in each case. It is therefore impossible to determine the effect of occupational exposure on bronchial reactivity.
* Specific bronchial provocation test
The specific bronchial provocation test is considered by most authors to be the "gold standard" for confirming or refuting the diagnosis of PA [6,9, 110,111].
The principle of this test is to have the patient inhale increasing doses of the molecule in question without reaching an irritating level. The positivity of specific bronchial provocation tests can be assessed by various techniques (FEV1, flow-volume curve, airway resistance) immediately after exposure, every 15 minutes for the first hour, then every hour for 8 hours and in the event of the onset of symptoms. The occurrence of bronchoconstriction with a 20% reduction in FEV1 confirms the harmfulness of the agent tested [13]. D. Choudat et al. have suggested that in cases where the variation in FEV1 is less than 20%, the results should be compared with the variations observed during the lactose test to avoid false negative results [112]. Beta-2 adrenergic bronchodilators and ipatropium bromide should be stopped 8 hours and theophylline 48 or 72 hours before the test, although they may be continued if spirometric variability is too great. The inhaled steroids sodium cromoglycate and sodium nedocromil should be continued, but only taken on the evening of each test day, at the same total dose, to avoid exacerbation of asthma due to discontinuation of treatment [113].
This test finds these indications mainly:[6]
- In the etiological diagnosis of PA induced by new substances.
- In diagnosing the causative agent in cases of exposure to several asthma-inducing substances.
- When other investigations are unavailable (skin tests, specific IgE assays) or uninterpretable (iterative measurements of PEF) or inconsistent.
This method requires certain precautions: [8]

- Exclusion of patients at risk (severe obstructive syndrome, cardiac problems or major associated pathologies, history of severe asthma, severe HRBNS)
- Carrying out the test in a hospital environment in the presence of trained staff.

This method, although considered a reference, has certain limitations: [6, 9, 109]

- Possibility of false negatives (incorrect identification of the causative agent, exposure to concentrations that are too low and/or for too short a time, tests carried out after prolonged eviction with loss of sensitivity to the causative agent).
- Possibility of false positive results (bronchial obstruction due to cessation of treatment, bronchospasm induced by forced exhalation manoeuvres)
- High cost.
- Difficult to put into practice.
- Lack of standardisation for most substances responsible for PA
- Contraindications: Severe obstructive ventilatory disorder (FEV1 less than 60% of predicted value) or unstable asthma (FEV1 variations greater than 12% during the "control" test).

In our study, TPS was carried out on 4 patients (Isocyanate, IRIKO wood, flour). The test was positive in each case and the diagnosis of PA was retained in all four cases.

4.2.3.2. Immunological tests

The immunological diagnosis of AP is only of interest when it involves an Ig E-dependent mechanism [6]. It demonstrates the existence of Ig E sensitisation mediated either by skin tests (prick test) or by in vitro measurement of specific Ig E (radio allergosorbent test or RAST) [109]. A positive skin test and/or specific Ig E assay indicates sensitisation, but does not provide proof that the respiratory symptoms observed are related to sensitisation [7].

Immunological tests are useful mainly for ruling out the diagnosis of PA, as their negative predictive value is close to 100%. However, they are of little help in confirming the existence of PA, as their positive predictive value is 75%.

. Immunological tests are commercially available for the HPM protein substances most frequently implicated in PA, such as cereals, natural latex, enzymes and laboratory animal allergens [109].

* Specific skin tests (SST) :

SCTs have the advantage of being a simple, rapid, inexpensive and completely harmless method [114]. Prick skin tests are more sensitive than ELISA serological tests [13].

Their use is generally straightforward for the most frequently implicated allergens of animal or plant origin, such as flour, latex and a-amylase, but they have no place in the diagnosis of PA caused by MPF agents [101].

According to the literature, the sensitivity of TCS for protein substances is excellent, while their specificity is fairly variable [109].

In our study, the results found were not very consistent with those found in the literature, and the specificity of TCS was 100% better than the sensitivity (71.4%) (positive predictive value 100%; negative predictive value 50%).

* Specific Ig E

The assay of specific Ig E may be the only element in the immunological diagnosis of AP, or it may supplement the investigation already carried out using skin tests.

The demonstration of specific Ig E is useful in demonstrating the existence of an Ig E-mediated immunological response to PMH agents [115].

The specific Ig E assay has the advantage of being a safe method [6]. It is available for the majority of occupational HPM allergens, in particular flour, latex, alpha amylase, proteolytic enzymes and laboratory animals. It is only possible for a very limited number of chemical allergens such as isocyanates, acid anhydrides or formaldehyde [101].

Some authors have shown that the concentration of specific Ig E decreases slowly after cessation of exposure: Rosemary D. Tee et al. have shown that the serum level of specific Ig E directed against Isocyanate decreases progressively from the thirtieth day following total eviction of the allergen [115].

Beach et al. found an average specific Ig E sensitivity of 73.3% and a specificity of 79% for PMH agents, whereas the sensitivity was 31% and the specificity 89% for MPF agents [116].

In our study, the sensitivity of specific Ig E was 75% and the sensitivity 50% (PPV 90%; NPV 25%).

The list of pneumallergens for which the specific Ig E assay is available in our university hospital centre is currently restricted to 21 reagents capable of detecting sensitisation to plant, animal and mould allergens.

5. Diagnostic strategy

The diagnostic strategy for HA involves three stages (Figure 24):

* Confirming the existence of asthma
* Asserting the occupational origin of asthma
* Identify the cause.

It follows clearly structured stages:

1) The first stage is based on anamnesis: a compatible clinical history (the notion of symptoms suggestive of work-related asthma) and exposure to possible causal agents.

In practice, any asthma that develops in an adult at the same time as occupational exposure to agents known to be likely to induce asthma should raise the possibility of PA.

2) The second stage: confirmation of asthma by EFR including pharmacological tests.

3) The third stage: demonstration of sensitisation to an occupational allergen by prick test or RAST.

4) The fourth stage: the demonstration of variations in functional parameters as a function of variations in exposure, possibly combined with the demonstration of variations in eosinophil levels in induced sputum or on specific bronchial provocation tests.

When it is not possible to monitor PEF or FEV1 longitudinally, or when the patient's cooperation is deemed insufficient, a specific bronchial provocation test should be encouraged, particularly for MPF substances.

The diagnosis of ***bronchial irritation*** syndrome (BIS) is based on the following criteria [111].

1) No previous respiratory symptoms.
2) Exposure to gas, smoke or vapours with irritating properties in high concentrations.
3) Symptoms begin within 24 hours of exposure and persist for at least 3 months.
4) Presence of symptoms reminiscent of asthma, with cough, dyspnoea and wheezing.
5) Objective evidence of bronchial asthma.
6) Exclusion of any other respiratory condition

No cases of SIB were recorded during our study. This may be explained by the fact that this entity was reported as an accident at work.

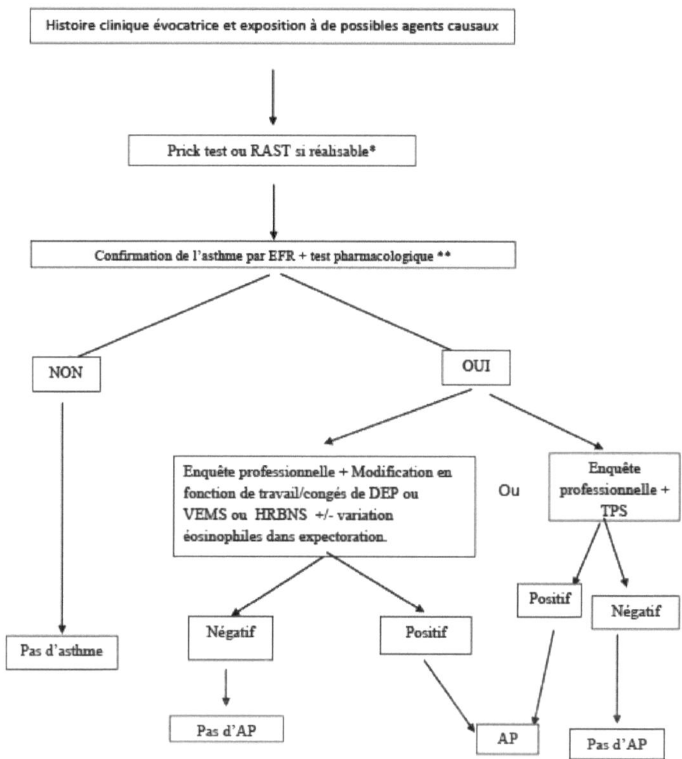

Figure 24: Algorithm for diagnosing PA [101].

*A negative test with an HPM allergen practically eliminates the responsibility of this allergen** The test must be carried out during a period of professional activity.

6. Differential diagnosis

Several pathological entities occurring in the workplace can mimic bronchial asthma. They must be distinguished from PA because of their different medico-legal management. These include: [111]

6.1. Asthma aggravated by work:

This is asthma that exists prior to work activity and whose symptoms worsen in the workplace (more frequent or more severe asthma attacks and/or increased medication required to achieve satisfactory asthma control during work periods) [114].

The specific bronchial provocation test is the most discriminating test, positive in PA and negative in work-aggravated asthma. Longitudinal monitoring of PEF and sequential study of the eosinophil count in induced sputum represent an interesting alternative [7].

6.2. Eosinophilic bronchitis

Eosinophilic bronchitis presents with a chronic cough, sputum, dyspnoea and rarely wheezing. It is distinguished from asthma by the absence of OVT and bronchial hyperreactivity [117].

6.3. Bronchiolitis

Bronchiolitis is an inflammatory disease of the bronchioles. Clinically, bronchiolitis is characterised by the development of exertional dyspnea and obstructive pulmonary dysfunction (OVP), which is not very responsive to bronchodilators. Formal diagnosis is then made on histological analysis of surgical lung samples [118].

6.4. Hypersensitivity pneumonitis

Hypersensitivity pneumonitis (HSP) is a pulmonary granulomatosis of immuno-allergic mechanism due to chronic inhalation of organic or chemical antigens, which is encountered mainly in the occupational environment [119]. The diagnosis of PHS is based on the demonstration of systemic signs absent in asthma, a reduction in diffusion capacity (DLCO) with or without a restrictive ventilatory syndrome, suggestive radiological abnormalities, the presence of lymphocytic alveolitis on BAL and compatible imaging (existence of nodules with blurred contours and/or bilateral ground-glass opacities on CT) [111].

6.5. Vocal cord dysfunction :

During attacks, vocal cord dysfunction is manifested by coughing, shortness of breath and, more rarely, hoarseness, dysphonia, chest tightness and difficulty swallowing [120]. Differential diagnosis with asthma, which is often difficult, is made by direct or indirect laryngeal fibroscopy or, better still, video-laryngoscopy, which reveals paradoxical closure of the vocal cords during the respiratory cycle of the front two-thirds, with persistent opening of a posterior laryngeal rhombus [111,120].

7. Support

7.1. Medical care

7.1.1. Elimination of the causative agent

Several authors have shown that early elimination of the allergen is the only effective method for hoping for a disappearance of the disease or a reduction in symptoms [47, 44, 96,121].

The earlier the eviction and the more moderate the symptoms, the better the progression of asthmatic disease [94].

Early eviction is therefore essential, especially as even with well-administered medical treatment, continued exposure to the incriminating agent leads to a progressive worsening of functional thoracic symptoms and a deterioration in

respiratory function [47].
However, even early and total cessation of exposure to occupational aerocontaminants is not always associated with an improvement in asthma, and symptoms may persist. Venables *et al.* showed that in a 6-year follow-up of patients with PA who were no longer exposed to the allergen, 90% showed an improvement in their symptoms, 72% were still on medication and reported symptoms during the last 3 months, and 40% to 73% reported limitations in their daily activities [121]. This may be explained by the persistence of HRBNS long after eviction [122].
Stopping exposure is often achieved at the cost of serious social consequences [123, 124,125]. Reducing exposure by transferring to a less exposed position in the same company, improving working conditions or using personal protective equipment is therefore an alternative worth considering [91].
Twelve patients in our series opted to stop work an average of 5.6 years after the onset of the first symptoms.

7.1.3. Pharmacological treatment :

Medical treatment of PA is often necessary, but should not replace preventive measures, especially environmental control. If exposure cannot be eliminated, or if symptoms persist despite the cessation of all contact with the offending molecule, therapeutic efforts should be undertaken to avoid or minimise the late asthmatic response [13]. Some authors state that even after removal of the agents responsible for PA, drug treatment is often still necessary [126].
Pharmacological treatment for patients with PA does not differ from the treatment of asthma in general [5, 13, 91, 126,127]. It must be adapted to the severity of the symptoms and is essentially based on a combination of bronchodilator and corticosteroid treatments [6].
Anti-histamine drugs should be used in the same way as for non-work-related asthma [91].
A longitudinal study of subjects who remained exposed to the causative agent of their disease suggested that treatment with inhaled corticoids and long-acting beta-mimetics could prevent deterioration in respiratory function [128]. However, two studies show that if workers remain exposed to the causal agent, whether red cedar [129] or various high and low molecular weight allergens [124], drug treatment does not prevent deterioration in lung function.
Nevertheless, another study has shown that the addition of inhaled corticosteroids to the cessation of exposure leads to a modest but significant improvement in asthma symptoms, quality of life and non-specific bronchial reactivity [130]. The benefits are greater if treatment is started early after diagnosis [91].

In our study, 20 patients were treated with pharmacological therapy. Ten of these patients, despite being completely allergen-free, still had asthma symptoms requiring background treatment.

7.1.4. Specific immunotherapy

Specific immunotherapy consists of the discontinuous administration of increasing doses of an allergen vaccine to an allergic patient with the aim of reducing symptoms and the drug requirements necessary to control the disease during subsequent allergen exposure [131].

There are very few studies of immunotherapy in HA [132]. The best documented trials concern subcutaneous immunotherapy in health professionals allergic to latex [133] or sublingual immunotherapy [134].

A few studies have shown some efficacy of immunotherapy in asthma caused by flour and laboratory animal allergens [121].

Recently, latex desensitisation has been performed in 9 patients, but the occurrence of systemic effects does not allow this type of treatment to be considered, at least in its current form, as an alternative to preventive methods [133]. According to J.Ameille et al., specific immunotherapy should not be used in PA (grade B recommendation) [91].

7.2. Medical and legal aspects

7.2.1. Declaration

7.2.1.1. In the world

* In Quebec

PA is a notifiable disease (MADO). Doctors are legally obliged to report MADOs to health and social services agencies [12].

* In the UNITED States:

PA is included in the list of *Sentinel Health Events (Occupational)* (SHE(O)). SHE(O) are work-related diseases that indicate the need to improve preventive measures for those exposed [135].

Several countries have official PA declaration systems:

* Finland: [21,26] the Finnish Institute of Occupational Health (FIOH) has set up a register to assess the exact incidence of PA.
* Germany: All doctors have a legal duty to report new cases of HA to the health insurance fund (Berufsgenossenschaft) [136].
* Belgium: The Fonds des maladies professionnelles (FMP) is responsible for medical expertise in the recognition of occupational diseases according to a list system [137].
* Italy: the medico-legal criteria required for the diagnosis and declaration of PA are based on the degree of bronchial obstruction on spirometry and HRBNS and the need for medication [138].

* Sweden: The Swedish Register of Reported Occupational Diseases (SRROD) collects all reports and complaints from employees concerning an occupational disease [139].

* In New Zealand: The Department of Labour Notifiable Occupational Disease System collects notifications of new cases of occupational pathology and identifies the substances involved [140].

In addition to these official PA reporting systems, other systems based on voluntary reporting by doctors have been set up in various countries with the aim of gaining a more exhaustive understanding of the incidence of PA.

* in England: the SWORD system (Surveillance of Work Related and Occupational Respiratory Disease): founded in 1989, its aim is to obtain a global record of all new cases of occupational respiratory diseases, including OI [141].

* In the West Midlands region of the United Kingdom: the SHIELD project: this system collects cases of PA reported by respirologists in the Midland Thoracic Society Research Group and by occupational physicians in the region [28].

* In the United States: the SENSOR (Sentinel Event Notification) programme System for Occupational Risks): its aim is to recognise and identify the agents responsible for OI in order, in a second stage, to propose investigations and preventive interventions in the workplace [29].

* In Italy: the PRIORITY system was set up in 1996. This system collects all identifications of new cases of HA by clinical centres comprising doctors specialising in allergology, pneumology and occupational medicine [30].

* In France :

The ONAP was set up in 1996 by the Societe de pneumologie de langue frangaise (SPLF) and the Societe frangaise de medecine du travail (SFMT). Its main aim is to determine as exhaustively as possible the number of new cases of PA [31].

7.2.1.2. In Tunisia :

Whatever the sector of activity, any worker suffering from an occupational illness which has been diagnosed by a doctor must notify the last employer by means of a declaration (special form) and an initial descriptive medical certificate (CMI). The latter informs the Caisse Nationale d'Assurance Maladie (CNAM) or the central commission of the prime minister (for the public sector) within five working days of the date on which the illness was first diagnosed.

The employer must notify the CNAM within three working days of being notified, and the local labour inspectorate.

After receiving the opinion of the recognition committee, the CNAM then grants the patient who has received a favourable opinion full cover for the medical check-ups and all types of medical check-ups and treatment prescribed. It should be noted that the patient is not obliged to provide proof of the relationship between his illness and his occupation: he benefits from the presumption of imputability and it is up to the CNAM to provide proof to the contrary if the occupational nature of the illness is rejected [141].

7.2.2. Repair

7.2.2.1. In the world

In France, asthma is listed in the tables of occupational diseases, which have three columns: the description of the disease "asthma as determined by respiratory function tests, relapsing in the event of new exposure to the risk or confirmed by test", the period for which the disease is covered (7 days) and the occupational exposure. If the causative agent is listed in one of the tables and if the criteria are met, asthma is recognised by presumption of origin. On the other hand, if the OE corresponds to a substance not listed in the tables, or if the criteria are not met, the case is examined by the CRRMP (Comite Regional de Reconnaissance des Maladies Professionnelles - Regional Committee for the Recognition of Occupational Diseases), law of 27.01.1993, paragraph 3. This must establish whether there is a direct relationship between occupational exposure and asthma.

Recognition of an occupational disease authorises free treatment and provides a daily allowance to compensate for salary in the event of absence from work and, in the event of sequelae, a rate of permanent partial disability (IPP). Unfortunately, declaring an occupational disease often exposes the worker to loss of employment [6].

7.2.22. In Tunisia

Compensation for asthma as an occupational disease is provided for in the tables set out in law 94/28. Some twenty tables are concerned by OA (Table XXX). In our series, the claim was made under tables 33, 36, 42, 44bis, 49, 53, 54, 56, 57 and 58.

In terms of compensation, there is an "indicative scale of permanent disability resulting from the after-effects of accidents at work and occupational diseases" which, under the heading of the respiratory system, provides for three degrees of impairment of respiratory function: mild, moderate and severe respiratory insufficiency [143].

The factors used to assess the deficit are dyspnea, chest X-ray data, basic spirometry data (vital capacity and Tiffeneau ratio) and signs of secondary cardiac complications. These assessment criteria, which are well suited to the evaluation of pneumoconiosis, are not adapted to the evaluation of occupational asthma [19].

Table XXX: Agents responsible for OI and the corresponding occupational disease table numbers

Occupational disease table number	***Etiological agent***
4	Cobalt and its mineral compounds
6	Nickel and its compounds
7	Chromium and its compounds
25	Aliphatic and alicyclic amines
28	Formaldehyde and its polymers
29	Furfural and furfuryl alcohol
33	Aromatic amines and their derivatives
34	Phenylhydrazine
42	Organic isocyanates
43	Vinyl chloride monomer
44bis	Allergic occupational diseases caused by latex (or natural rubber) proteins.
47	Penicillins and their salts and cephalosporins
49	Enzymes
52	Macrolides
53	Plant textile dusts
54	Woods and cork
56	Cereals and flour
57	Other plant dusts
58	Other agents responsible for allergic respiratory diseases

To facilitate the diagnosis of 1'AP a new guide has been implemented. This document sets out a new scientific approach to identifying cases of PA. Practitioners can refer to this report, presented in the quarterly review of general information published by the ISST (Institut de sante et de securite au travail) number 24 of January 2003, which sets out for each type of asthma the investigations to be carried out, the prognosis to be established and the medication to be used according to the degree of severity observed.

8. Medical, socio-economic and professional consequences

8.2. Medical consequences

The evolution of the respiratory state of a subject with PA is highly variable, depending on several factors: [16]

* Land :

- Initial atopic condition
- Smoking adds

* The allergen :

- Level or concentration of exposure or allergenic load
- Its ubiquitous nature
- Its irritating action

- Type of allergen (some, such as isocyanates, cause more severe asthma)
* Concomitant exposure to other irritants
* Exhibition time
* Early eviction

Some studies have shown that the disease can progress towards recovery if the eviction is definitive and real [142].

However, in spite of complete eviction, it is recognised that a high number of patients with PA have long-term symptoms [6, 13, 143].

On average, all the studies published in the literature report identical data: more than 50% of patients removed from their occupational environment retain symptoms and HRBNS. The substances most frequently studied were isocyanates, red cedar, rosin, snow crab proteins, etc. [144].

The persistence of symptoms is thought to be linked to the persistence of HRBNS [122].

The factors determining this pejorative evolution have been studied [145]: they are most often

* Patients with a long period of exposure at the time of diagnosis of PA
* A prolonged period of symptoms
* Clear impairment of functional tests
* A severe HRBNS.

Severe cases are exceptional, but 10 cases of fatal PA have been reported in the literature [146].

In the course of our study, 12 patients opted to stop work (or to avoid the allergen altogether) a few years after the onset of their symptoms (at an average of 5.6 years). Ten of them reported a deterioration in their quality of life, with persistent respiratory symptoms limiting their physical activity in spite of well-monitored medical treatment, and a drop in their income.

8.2. Socio-economic and professional consequences

Often, eviction is not possible or is incomplete, leading to dismissal due to unfitness for the job, and then, when this is possible, to redeployment. Stopping work is often refused by the patient, who prefers to live with his or her disability and refuses to declare an occupational disease (despite the social security cover available in France, compensation is not enough to make up for the financial loss; almost half of patients lose their jobs and a third remain exposed to the risk) [6].

Dismissal comes at the cost of serious socio-economic consequences (loss or reduction of income) [123]. This was the case for 12 patients in our series.

9. Prevention

9.1. Primary prevention

Primary prevention includes all actions designed to reduce the risk of new cases appearing, and therefore to reduce the incidence of a disease in a population.
In the case of the PA, this prevention has several components:

* Avoiding people at high risk of developing asthma in their future profession

The predictive value of atopy in PA is low. There is therefore no justification for recommending that people with atopy should be excluded from at-risk professions (bakers, laboratory workers, etc.), but rather for promoting information about the risks and the importance of regular medical surveillance in people with atopy [147,148].

* Training and informing employees about the risk and means of prevention [147].

* Collective and individual prevention

This refers to all the technical measures used to eliminate or reduce exposure to a potentially sensitising agent:

* Collective prevention: Several actions have been proposed: replacement of the offending product or component, working in a closed cup or closed circuit, automation of manufacturing processes, general ventilation of premises, vacuum extraction, humidification of premises, frequent cleaning of premises, etc. [147,148].

* Individual prevention: This must complement collective prevention. It essentially involves raising awareness of respiratory protection devices (filtering and insulating masks) [147].

9.2. Secondary prevention

Secondary prevention, as defined by the World Health Organisation (WHO), is all measures aimed at the early detection of diseases, with the aim of discovering them at a stage when they can be treated. In the context of the PA, this means selective screening for high-risk groups, in particular during pre-recruitment and periodic medical check-ups.

This screening should include a questionnaire, a physical examination and an assessment of lung function [147]. For subjects exposed to MPF products, the combined use of the questionnaire and the bronchial reactivity test is recommended as a means of detecting subjects in the early stages of PA.

9.3. Tertiary prevention

The medical treatment of PA is no different from that for allergic asthma [5].

The best treatment for PA is early and definitive eviction.

5 CONCLUSION

PA has become the most common work-related respiratory disease. Moreover, epidemiological data suggest that 10% of adult asthma can be attributed to occupational activity.

This disease affects a young, economically active population, and thus has a considerable socio-economic cost. The impact of this disease could be considerably minimised by appropriate preventive measures.

We conducted a retrospective descriptive study of all cases of PA reported to the CNAM regional offices over an eight-year period from 01/01/2002 to 31/12/2009.

The aims of our study were to investigate the frequency of PA in southern Tunisia, to establish its diagnostic strategy, to describe the epidemiological features of the subjects affected, the etiological factors, in particular the main trades involved, and to specify the therapeutic, evolutionary, preventive and medico-legal aspects of the disease.

For the collection of data, we consulted the patient files filed in the archives of the pneumology department, the medical and administrative files of patients declared for PA (initial medical certificate (CMI), para-clinical assessment, etc.) collected from the regional offices of the CNAM in Sfax, and the data from the occupational survey conducted by the CNAM for all declared cases.

All clinical and para-clinical data were recorded on a synoptic sheet.

- In total, fifty-nine cases of PA were collected in our study, i.e. 7.3 cases/year. This result may underestimate the actual number of PA cases. This underestimate is due to the retrospective nature of our study.
- Our population was predominantly male (44 cases or 74.5%). The sex ratio is thus estimated at 2.93.
- The average age of our patients is 42+/- 9 years.
- More than half the cases originated in the city of Sfax (54.2% of cases); the incidence of this disease in this region is estimated at 40/100,000 workers.
- Most of the patients reported (40 patients) were manual workers employed by companies in the secondary sector, with the agri-food and textile industries at the top of the list.
- The diagnosis of AP was based on two fundamental steps: firstly, the diagnosis of asthma, and secondly, confirmation of its occupational nature.

1) To establish the diagnosis of asthma, an assessment was carried out including

> a detailed interrogation which provided the following data

- Familial atopy was noted in only one case, while personal atopy was found in 13 patients.
- Functional symptoms were dominated by wheezing (44 cases, 74.5%) and

chronic dry cough (13 cases, 22%).

- Associated atopic symptoms were found in 19 patients.

> A somatic examination was found to be normal in almost half the patients (26 patients, or 44%). In addition, sibilant and snoring noises were noted in 37.2% and 11.8% of patients respectively. Skin, otorhinological and ophthalmological examination data were not detailed in our files.

> The paraclinical assessment includes :

- Biological analysis (CBC and total IgE assay): hyper-eosinophilia was noted in 7 patients and elevated total IgE was found in 11 patients.
- A radiological assessment (a standard chest X-ray was carried out for all patients and a sinus X-ray was carried out for 3 patients)
- Functional assessment: spirometry, the reports of which could only be recovered for 48 patients, revealed an obstructive syndrome in 32 patients (severe obstructive pulmonary disease in 14 patients). Significant reversibility in a beta-2 mimetic test was sought and achieved in 3 of the 48 patients with OVT. A non-specific bronchial provocation test with metacholine performed on 10 patients with completely normal spirometry was positive in 10 of them.

2) Confirmation of the professional nature of asthma was based on

> Questioning data:

- The average length of exposure to occupational risk was 14+/- 7 years.

- The average time to onset of the first symptoms in relation to the date of recruitment was 9.33 years +/- 6.8 years. It should be noted that the onset of symptoms was earlier for atopic subjects than for non-atopic subjects.
- The average duration of symptoms before the first consultation is estimated at 4.42 ± 5 years, with extremes ranging from a few months to 24 years.
- Symptomatology related to occupational exposure, with respiratory problems improving during weekly rest periods and/or annual leave and worsening during periods of activity, was reported by 25 patients (42.3%).

> Paraclinical assessment data

- An assay of specific Ig E directed against the incriminating agent. This test revealed the presence of specific immunoglobulin directed against methyl methacrylate (one case), cereals and flour (3 cases), latex (2 cases), isocyanate (3 cases) and phenol nitrate derivatives (1 case).
- A staged spirometry consisting of a spirometry at the time of occupational exposure and a second spirometry 7 days after eviction was used to confirm the occupational nature of the asthma in 10 patients, demonstrating an improvement in the obstructive syndrome without any treatment.
- A specific bronchial provocation test was carried out in 4 patients. The allergens used were flour, wood and humidity.

> Data from the workplace study carried out by an agent appointed by the CNAM. The aim of this study is to determine the actual exposure to the suspected allergen by means of questioning, as well as the working conditions during handling of the incriminated substance and the possible use of protective equipment. In our study, this investigation was carried out for all reported cases. It confirmed exposure to the suspected etiological agent in 50 patients, i.e. 84.7% of reported cases.

- The main causal agents were flour (10 cases), isocyanates (10 cases), textile dusts (5 cases), wood and cork (5 cases).
- Once the diagnosis of AP has been established, the treating physician, in collaboration with the occupational physician, proceeds with the declaration. In the context of our study, this was done essentially under 3 tables: table No. 42 relating to isocyanates; table No. 56 relating to cereals and flour; table No. 58: corresponding to other agents responsible for allergic respiratory diseases.
- The 59 cases of AP declared are systematically examined by a specialised commission of the CNAM. The legal consequences were as follows

- Recognition as an occupational disease in 38 cases
- Rejection in 21 cases for medical reasons (8 cases), administrative reasons (10 cases), medical and administrative reasons (3 cases).

- For recognised cases, in addition to covering the costs of clinical and paraclinical investigations, the compensation procedure includes a permanent cash benefit awarded on the basis of the rate of permanent partial disability (IPP) set by a specialised medical committee within the CNAM. The average rate of PPI awarded to patients receiving compensation was 24%.

- There are two main aspects to the treatment of AP
- Eviction by voluntary redundancy (12 patients) or transfer of post (3 cases)
- One medical treatment for 20 patients.
- AP has serious medical and social consequences, and ten of the patients (16.9%) who have stopped working report a deterioration in their quality of life due to the persistent deterioration in their respiratory condition, which limits their daily activities, and a drop in their income.
- AP is one of the most common occupational respiratory diseases, but it is often underestimated and/or under-reported. Given the potential seriousness of this disease, which is dominated by the risk of chronic respiratory insufficiency and the serious socio-economic consequences, it is essential to optimise the means of prevention, particularly primary prevention, and the means of treating it by developing better collaboration between the various occupational health and safety authorities. collaboration between the various the occupational physician, the pneumo-allergologist, the insurer, the employee and the employer.

6 BIBLIOGRAPHY

1. **Vandenplas O, Larbanois A, Bugli C, Kampeneers E, Nemery B**. Epidemiology of occupational asthma in Belgium. Rev Mal Respir 2005; 22: 421-30.

2. **Caldeira RD, Bettiol H, Barbieri M A, Terra-Filho J, Garcia C A, Vianna E A.** Prevalence and risk factors for work related asthma in young adults. Occup Environ Med 2006; 63:694- 99.

3. **Birba E, Donnay C, Pauli G.** Current aspects of occupational asthma and rhinitis. Revue fran^aise d'allergologie et d'immunologie clinique 2003; 43: 401- 07.

4. **Chaari N, Amri C, Khalfallah T, Alaya A, Abdallah B, Harzallah L et al**. Rhinitis and asthma related to cotton dust exposure in clothing apprentices. Revue des maladies respiratoirtes 2009 ; 26 :29- 36.

5. **Pauli G, Kopferschmitt-Kubler M-C.** Asthme professionnel strategie diagnostique et prise en charge : Le point de vue du pneumologue. Rev Mal Respir 2006; 23: 89-90.

6. **Kopferschmitt- Kubler M C, Popin E, Pauli G.** Diagnosis and management of occupational asthma. Revue Mal Respir 2008; 25 ; 999-1012.

7. **Ameille.J.** Asthma aggravated by work: is it occupational asthma? Revue fran^aise d'allergologie 2009; 49: 122-24.

8. **Vandenplas O, Malo J-L**. Definitions and types of work-related asthma: a nosological approach. Eur Respir J 2003; 21: 706- 12.

9. **Pauli G, Bessot J-C, Vervloet D, Ameille J.** Investigations diagnostiques de l'asthme professionnel, necessite et limites (The need for and limits of diagnostic test for professional asthma). Rev Mal Respir 2002; 19: 289-91.

10. **Ameille J, Larbanois A, Descatha A, Vandenplas O.** Epidemiology and etiology of occupational asthma. Rev Mal Respir 2006; 26: 726-40.

11. **Moira Chan - Yeung.** Occupational asthma - the past 50 years. Can Respir J 2004; 11: 21-6

12. **Arif AA, Whitehead LW, Delclos GL, Tortolero SR, Lee ES.** Prevalence and risk factors of work related asthma by industry among United States workers: data from the third national health and nutrition examination survey (1988-94). *Occup Envlron Med* 2002; 59: 505-11

13. **Deschamps F, Deschamps- boulanger S.** Occupational asthma in 1997. Rev fr Allergol 1997; 37: 3.

14. **Blanc P.** Occupational asthma in a national disability survey. Chest 1987; 92: 613-17.

15. **Kogevinas Manolis, Maria Anto Josep, Sunyer Jordi, Tobias Aurelio, Kromhout Hans, Burney Peter.** Occupational asthma in Europe and other industrialised areas: a population-based study. Lancet 1999; 353 (9166): 1750-4.

16. **Landric M, Demoly P.** Asthmes professionnels (Occupational Asthma). Revue fran^aise d'allergologie et d'immunologie clinique 2006; 46: 51-5.

17. **Meyer J D, Holt DL, Chery N M, Mc Donald J C.** Surveillance of work- related and occupational respiratory disease in the UK. SWORD 98 occupational medicine 1999; 49(8): 485-89.

18. **Dahmoul M.** Asthme professionnel : Epidemiologie, facteurs de risque, aspects medico-legaux de l'AP - Analyse retrospective a propos de 244 cas colliges a la CNAM de la région du centre sur une periode de 9 ans. These medecine Sousse 2008/2009.

19. **Daly L, Nouaigui H, Hammadi M, Rammeh H, Ben laiba M.** L'asthme professionnel. Revue de la sante et securite au travail 2001; 19: 2-20.

20. **Yuriko Iwatsubo, Ellen Imbernon, Emeline Chabault, Jacques Ameille.** Surveillance epidemiologique des asthmes d'origine professionnelle : etude pilote avec l'Observatoire national des asthmes professionnels (Onap). Sante Travail 2007; 1-20.

21. **Kopferschmitt-Kubler, Romier-Borgnat S, Popin E, Port-Wasser C, Bessot J-C, Pauli G.** Les systemes de surveillance de l'asthme professionnel a travers le monde. Rev Fr

Allergol immunol Cln 2000; 40: 37480.

22. **Meredith S Nordman H**. Occupational asthma: measures of frequency from four countries. Thorax 1996; 51: 435-40

23. **Thimpont J, Paquier L, Dumortier P, Farr P, De Brouwer C, Strauss P et al**. Les missions du Fonds des Maladies Professionnelles. La sous- déclaration des cancers respiratoires professionnels, en particulier dus a l'amiante. Rev Med Brux. 2009 ; 30 : 318-25.

24. **Diar Bakerly N, Moore V C, Vellore A D, Jaakkola M S, Robertson A S, Burge P S.** Fifteen-year trends in occupational asthma: data from the Shield surveillance scheme. Occupational Medicine 2008;58:169-74.

25. **Walls C, Crane J, Gillies J, Wilsher M, Wong C**. Occupational asthma cases notified to OSH from 1996 to 1999. New Zealand Med J 1997; 110: 246-9.

26. **Kari Reijula, Tari Haahtela, Timo Klaukka, Jorma Rantanen.** Incidence of Occupational Asthma and Persistent Asthma in Young Adults Has Increased in Finland. Chest 1996;110 : 58-61.

27. **Beckett W S.** The epidemiology of occupational asthma. Eur Respir J 1994; 7: 161-4.

28. **Gannon P F G, Sherwood Burge P.** The SHIELD scheme in the West Midlands Region,United Kingdom. British Journal of Industril Medicine 1993; 50:791-96.

29. **Baker L.** Sentinel Event Notification System for Occupational Risks. American Journal of Public Health 1989; 79: 18-20.

30. **Bena A, D'Errico A, Mirabelli D.** A system for the active surveillance of occupational bronchial asthma: the results of 2 years of activity of the PRIOR program. Medicina del Lavoro 1990; 90: 556-71.

31. **Kopferschmitt-Kubler M C, Popin E, Vervloet D, Ameille J, Pauli G.** L'observatoire national des asthmes professionnels (The National Occupational Asthma Registry). Revue fran^aise d'allergologie et d'immunologie clinique 2003; 43: 6-12.

32. **Popin E, Kopferschmitt-Kubler M C, Gonzales M, Brom M, Flesch F, Pauli G.** L'asthme professionnel en Alsace : quelques particularites regionales Resultats de l'intensification locale de l'ONAP en 2001-2002. Rev Mal Respir 2008; 25: 806-13.

33. **Haddar M, Kaced N, Korichi S, Alloula R.** Prevalence of occupational asthma: a survey of occupational sectors. Archives des Maladies Professionnelles et de l'Environnement 2004; 65: 541-50.

34. **Fishwick D, Pearce N, D'Souza W, Lewis S, Town I, Armstrong R et al.** Occupational asthma in New Zealanders: a population based study. Occupational and Environmental Medicine 1997; 54:301-6.

35. **Karjalainen A, Kurppa K, Martikainen R, Karjalainen J, Klaukka T.** Exploration of asthma risk by occupation: extended analysis of an incidence study of the Finnish population. Scand J Work Environ Health 2002; 28:4957.

36. **Nicole Le Moual, Susan M. Kennedy, Francine Kauffmann**. Occupational exposures and asthma in 14,000 adults from the general population. Am J Epidemiol 2004; 160: 1108-16.

37. **Ng TP, Hong CY, Goh LG, Wong ML, Koh KT, Ling SL.** Risk of asthma associated with occupations in a community- based case - control study. Am J Ind Med 1994; 25: 709-18.

38. **Jouni J. K. Jaakkola, Ritva Piipari, Maritta S. Jaakkola.** Occupation and Asthma: A Population-based Incident Case-Control Study. American Journal of Epidemiology 2003; 158,981-7.

39. **Kopferschmitt-Kubler MC, Clalastreng-Crinquand A, Romier-Borgnat S, Popin E, Vervloet D.** Observatoire national des asthmes professionnels (ONAP) : derniers resultats. *Souffle* 1998, 26: 4-6.

40. **Johansson SGO, OB Hourihane J, Bousquet J, Bruijnzeel-Koomen C, Dreborg S, Haahtela T et al.** A revised nomenclature for allergy: An EAACI position statement from the EAACI nomenclature task force Allergy 2001; 56: 813-24.
41. **Denyse Gautrin, Herberto Ghezzo, Claire Infante-Rivard, Jean-Luc Malo.** Incidence and Determinants of Ig E-mediated Sensitization in Apprentices: A Prospective Study. Am J Respir Crit Care Med 2000; 162: 1222- 8.
42. **MALO J L**. What's new in occupational asthma? Revue fran^aise d'allergologie et d'immunologie clinique 1996; 36: 955-59.
43. **Lemiere C, Charpin D, Vervloet D.** Is atopy a risk factor for occupational asthma? Revue des maladies respiratoires 1995; 12: 231-9.
44. **Emil J, Bardana Jr.** Occupational asthma and related respiratory disorders. Disease a month 1995; 41: 145-99.
45. **Barnig C, Blay F.** Epidemiology of occupational respiratory allergies. Revue fran^aise d'allergologie 2009; 49: 116-21.
46. **Botham P A, Davies G E, Teasdale E L.** Allergy to laboratory animals: a prospective study of its incidence and of the influence of atopy on its development. British Journal of Industrial Medicine 1987; 44: 627-32.
47. **Mark S, Dykewicz MD, Winston-Salem NC.** Occupational asthma: Current concepts in pathogenesis, diagnosis, and management. J Allergy Clin Immunol 2009; 123: 519-28.
48. **Gianna Moscato, Olivier Vandenplas, Roy Gerth Van Wijk, Jean- Luc Malo, Luca Perfetti.** EAACI position paper on occupational rhinitis. Respiratory Research 2009; 10: 1-20.
49. **Siracusa A, Marabini A, Folletti I, Moscato G.** Smoking and occupational asthma. Clinical and Experimental Allergy 2006; 36: 577- 84.
50. **Katherine M Venables, Michael B Dally, Andrew J Nunn, Jane F Stevens, Richard Stephens, Neil Farrer et al.** Smoking and occupational allergy in workers in a platinum refinery. British Medical Journal 1989; 299: 939-42.
51. **Venables K M, Topping M D, Howe W, Luczynska C M, Hawkins R, Newman Taylor A J.** Interaction of smoking and atopy in producing specific IgE antibody against a hapten protein conjugate. British Medical Journal 1985; 290: 201-4.
52. **Moira Chan-Yeung.** Occupational Asthma. Environ Health Perspect 1995; 6: 249-52
53. **Monier S, Hemery M L, Demoly P, Dhivert-Donnadieu H.** Occupational asthma to wood dust. Revue fran^aise d'allergologie et d'immunologie clinique 2008; 48: 31-4.
54. **Zetterstrom O, Nordvall S L, Bjorksten B, Ahlstedt S, Stelander M.** Increased IgE antibody responses in rats exposed to tobacco smoke. Journal of allergy and clinical immunology 1985; 75: 594-8.
55. **Katherine M Venables, Upton J L, Rosemarie Hawkins E, Rosemary D Tee, Joan L Longbottom, Newman Taylor A J.** Smoking. Atopy and laboratory animal allergy. British Journal of Industrial Medicine 1988; 45: 66771.
56. **Calverley A E, Rees D, Dowdeswell R J, Linnett P J, Kielkowski D.** Platinum salt sensitivity in refinery workers: incidence and effects of smoking and exposure. Occupational and Environmental Medicine 1995; 52: 661-6.
57. **Bricard C, Floret E, Delecluse P, Boury E**. Non-specific bronchial hyperreactivity and methacholine provocation test. Lyon Pharmaceutique 2001; 52: 166-81.
58. **Gautrin D.** Epidemiology, risk factors and diagnosis of occupational asthma. Revue fran^aise d'allergologie et d'immunologie clinique1998; 38: 132- 40.
59. **Moira Chan-Yeung, Desjardins A.** Bronchial hyperresponsiveness and level of exposure in occupational asthma due to western red cedar (Thuja plicata): serial observations before and after development of symptoms. The American review of respiratory disease 1992; 146: 1606-9.

60. **Denyse Gautrin, Claire Infante-Rivard, Herberto Ghezzo, Jean- Luc Malo.** Incidence and Host Determinants of Probable Occupational Asthma in Apprentices Exposed to laboratory Animals. American journal of respiratory and critical care medicine 2001; 163: 899- 904.
61. **Bignon J S, Aron Y, Ju L Y, Kopferschmitt M C, Garnier R, Mapp C et al**. HLA class II alleles in isocyanate-induced asthma. American Journal of Respiratory and Critical Care Medicine 1994; 149: 71-5.
62. **Horne C, Quintana P J E, Keown P A, Dimich-Ward H, Chan-Yeung M.** Distribution of DRB1 and DQB1 HLA class II alleles in occupational asthma due to western red cedar. European Respiratory Journal 2000; 15: 911- 4.
63. **Balboni A, Baricordi O R, Fabbri L M, Gandini E, Ciaccia A, Mapp C E**. Association between toluene diisocyanate- induced asthma and DQB1 markers: a possible role for aspartic acid at position 57. European Respiratory Journal 1996; 9 : 207-10.
64. **Mapp Beghe, Balboni Zamorani, Padoan Jovine, Baricordi Fabbri.** Association between HLA genes and susceptibility to toluene diisocyanate- induced asthma. Clinical and Experimental Allergy 2000; 30 : 651-6.
65. **Hans-Peter Rihs, Tirze Barbalho-Krolls, Hermann Huber, Xaver Baur**. No evidence for the influence of HLA class II in alleles in isocyanate-induced asthma. American Journal of Industrial Medicine 1997; 32: 522-7.
66. **Jonathan A. Bernstein, Jennifer Munson, Zana L. Lummus, Kamaia Balakrishnan, George Leikauf.** T-cell receptor Vl3 gene segment expression in diisocyanate-induced occupational asthma. The Journal of Allergy and Clinical Immunology 1997; 99: 245 50.
67. **Beghe B, Padoan M, Moss CT, Barton SJ, Holloway JW, Holgate ST et al**. Lack of association of HLA class I genes and TNF alpha-308 polymorphism in toluene diisocyanate-induced asthma. Allergy 2004; 59: 614.
68. **Young RP, Barker RD, Pile KD, Cookson WO, Taylor AJ.** The association of HLA-DR3 with specific IgE to inhaled acid anhydrides. Am J Respir Crit Care Med 1995; 151: 219-221.
69. **Jones M G, Nielsen J, Welch, Harris, Welinder, Bensryd I et al.** Association of HLA-DQ5 and HLA-DR1 with sensitization to organic acid anhydrides. Clinical and Experimental Allergy 2004; 34: 812-6.
70. **Anthony J. Newman Taylor, Paul Cullinan, Penny A Lympany, Jessica M Harris, Robert J. Dowdeswell.** Interaction of HLA Phenotype and Exposure Intensity in Sensitization to Complex Platinum Salts. American Journal of Respiratory and Critical Care Medicine 1999; 160: 435-8.
71. **Hans-Peter Rihs, Zhiping Chen, Franziska Ruëff, Reinhold Cremer, Monika Raulf-Heimsoth, Xaver Baur et al.** HLA-DQ8 and the HLA-DQ8- DR4 haplotype are positively associated with the hevein-specific IgE immune response in health care workers with latex allergy. The Journal of Allergy and Clinical Immunology 2002; 110: 507-14.
72. **Hayley Jeal, Adrian Draper, Meinir Jones, Jessica Harris, Ken Welsh, Anthony Newman Taylor et al.** HLA associations with occupational sensitization to rat lipocalin allergens: A model for other animal allergies? The Journal of Allergy and Clinical Immunology 2003; 111: 795-9.
73. **Piirila Paivi, Wikman Harriet, Luukkonen Ritva, Kaaria Katja, Rosenberg Christina, Nordman Henrik et al.** Glutathione S-transferase genotypes and allergic responses to diisocyanate exposure. Pharmacogenetics 2001; 11: 437-45.
74. **Wikman H, Piirila P, Rosenberg C, Luukkonen R, Kaaria K, Nordman H et al.** N-Acetyltransferase genotypes as modifiers of diisocyanate exposure- associated asthma risk. Pharmacogenetics 2002; 12: 227-33.
75. **Cristina E Mapp, Anthony A Fryer, Nicoletta De Marzo, Valeria Pozzato, Michele**

Padoan, Piera Boschetto et al. Glutathione S-transferase GSTP1 is a susceptibility gene for occupational asthma induced by isocyanates. The Journal of Allergy and Clinical Immunology 2002; 109: 867-72.

76. **A Hollander, D Heederik, G Doekes.** Respiratory allergy to rats: exposureresponse relationships in laboratory animal workers. American Journal of Respiratory and Critical Care Medicine 1997; 155: 562-7.

77. **Remko Houba, Dick Heederik, Gert Doekes.** Wheat Sensitization and Work-related Symptoms in the Baking Industry Are Preventable An Epidemiologic Study. American journal of respiratory and critical care medicine 1998; 158: 1499-503.

78. **Houba R, Heederik DJ, Doekes G, Van Run PE.** Exposure -sensitization relationship for alpha-amylase allergens in the baking industry. American Journal of Respiratory and Critical Care Medicine 1996; 154: 130-6.

79. **Cullinan P, Lowson D, Nieuwenhuijsen MJ, Gordon S, Tee RD, Venables KM et al.** Work related symptoms, sensitisation, and estimated exposure in workers not previously exposed to laboratory rats. Occupational and Environmental Medicine 1994; 51: 589-92.

80. **Baur X, Chen Z, Allmers H.** Can a threshold limit value for natural rubber latex airborne allergens be defined. J Allergy Clin Immunol 1998; 101: 24-7.

81. **C.-Y. Li, E-C. Sung.** A review of the healthy worker effect in occupational epidemiology. Occup. Med 1999; 49: 225-9.

82. **Elms J, Fishwick D, Walker J, Rawbone R, Jeffrey P, Griffin P et al.** Prevalence of sensitisation to cellulase and xylanase in bakery workers. Occup Environ Med 2003; 60:802-4.

83. Enzyme-induced occupational asthma. INRS document pour le medecin du travail 2007; 112 ; 553-64.

84. **Jeebhay M F, Robins T G, Lehrer S B, Lopata A L.** Occupational seafood allergy: a review. Occup Environ Med 2001; 58: 553-62.

85. **Boeniger MF, Lummus ZL, Biagini RE, Bernstein DI, Swanson MC, Reed C et al.** Exposure to protein aeroallergens in egg processing facilities. Appl Occup Environ Hyg 2001 ; 16 : 660-70.

86. **Bessot J C, Blaumeiser M, Kopferschmitt M, Pauli G.** L'asthme professionnel en milieu agricole = Occupational asthma in a farming environment. Revue des maladies respiratoires 1996; 13: 205-16.

87. **Cristina E. Mapp, Piera Boschetto, Piero Maestrelli, Leonardo M. Fabbri.** Occupational Asthma. American Journal of Respiratory and Critical Care Medicine 2005; 172: 280-350.

88. **Mapp C E, Saetta M, Maestrelli P, Di Stefano A, Chitano P, Boschetto P et al.** Mechanisms and pathology of occupational asthma. Eur Respir J 1994; 7: 544-54.

89. **Lynda J Lombardo, John R. Balmes.** Occupational Asthma: A Review. Environmental Health Perspectives 2000; 108: 697-704.

90. **Sastre J, Vandenplas O, Park H S.** Pathogenesis of occupational asthma. Eur Respir J 2003; 22: 364-73.

91. **Taille C.** Adult asthma: diagnosis and treatment (excluding acute asthma). EMC-Medecine 2004; 1: 141-50.

92. **Marguet D, Michelet I, Couderc L, Lubrano M.** La crise d'asthme aiguë en pediatrie. Archives de Pediatrie 2009; 16: 505-7.

93. **Brimont G, Ricard-Selva C, Caubet Y, Moisan V, Dutau G.** Les prodromes de l'asthme: les identifier et mieux les utiliser. Rev Fr Allergol 1991; 31: 231-34.

94. Guidelines for the Diagnosis and Management of Asthma. National Heart, Lung, and Blood Institute National Asthma Education Prevention Program. Full Report 2007. 1-440.

95. A reminder about peak expiratory flow. Revue des maladies respiratoires 2005; 22: 85-6.

96. **Quanjer P H, Lebowitz M D, Gregg I, Miller M R, Pedersen O F.** Peak expiratory flow: conclusions and recommendations of a Working Party of the European Respiratory Society . Eur Respir J 1997; 10: 2-8.
97. L'asthme. Revue des Maladies Respiratoires 2002; 19: 25-9.
98. **Watelet J -B.** Rhinitis and asthma: one airway, one disease? Revue fran^aise d'allergologie et d'immunologie Clinique 2008; 48: 17-8.
99. **Rosenberg N.** Occupational asthma caused by rosin. Documents pour le medecin du Travail 2003; 94: 195-200.
100. **Susan M. Tarlo, Gary M. Liss, Paul D, Blanc.** How to diagnose and treat work-related asthma. Key messages for clinical practice from the American College of Chest Physicians Consensus Statement. Archives de Pologne medecine interne 2009; 119: 660-6
101. **Ameille J, Choudat D, Pairon J C, Pauli G, Perdrix A, Vandenplas O.** What are the interactions between allergic asthma and the occupational environment? Revue des maladies respiratoires 2007; 24: 52-67.
102. **Mairesse M, Ledent C.** Asthme et rhinite d'origine professionnelle cause par le sene ; Occupational asthma and rhinithis caused by senna. Revue fran^aise d'allergologie et d'immunologie clinique 2007; 47: 371-2.
103. **Rosenberg N.** Occupational respiratory allergies caused by wood dust. Doc Med Travail 2003; 96: 501-10.
104. **Surber R, Guberan M, Girard J P.** Allergies respiratoires aux poussières de bois, Cas cliniques et études epidemiologiques. Revue fran^aise Allergologie 1977; 17: 193-8.
105. **Malo J L, Lemiere C, Desjardins A, Cartier A.** Prevalence and intensity of rhinoconjunctivitis in subjects with occupational asthma. European Respiratory Journal 1997; 10: 1513-15.
106. **Moscato G, Godnic-Cvar J, Maestrelli P, Malo JL, Burge PS, Coifman R.** Subcommittee on Occupational Asthma of the European Academy of Allergy and Clinical Immunology. Statement on self-monitoring of peak expiratory flows in the investigation of occupational asthma. Eur Respir J 1995; 8: 160510.
107. **Jean-Luc Malo, Johanne Cote, Andre Cartier, Louis-Philippe Boulet, Jocelyne L'Archeveque, Moira Chan-Yeung.** How many times per day should peak expiratory flow rates be assessed when investigating occupational asthma? Thorax 1993; 48: 1211-7.
108. **Anees W, P.F. Gannon P F, Huggins V, Pantin C F A, Burge P S**. Effect of peak expiratory flow data quantity on diagnostic sensitivity and specificity in occupational asthma. Eur Respir J 2004; 23: 730- 4.
109. **Vandemplas O, Larbanois A, Delwiche J P**. Diagnostic approaches to occupational asthma. Rev Mal Respir 2002; *19:* 334-40.
110. **Cartier A, Malo J L.** Investigation and outcome of occupational asthma. Rev fr Allergol 1985; 25: 171-79.
111. **Ramon Orriols Martinez, Khalil Abu Shams, Enrique Alday Figueroa, Maria Jesus Cruz Carmona, Juan Bautista Galdiz Iturri, Isabel Isidro Montes et al**. Guidelines for Occupational Asthma. Arch Bronconeumol 2006; 42: 457-74.
112. **Choudat D, Martin J C, Fabries J F, Villette C, Dessanges J F.** Test de provocation bronchique specifique avec aerosols solides. Quantification des resultats. Revue des Maladies Respiratoires 2001; 18: 157-162.
113. **Vandenplas O, Malo JL.** Inhalational challenges with agents causing occupational asthma. *Eur Respir J* 1997, 10: 2612-29.
114. **Olivier Vandenplas, Frangoise Binard-Van Cangh, Andre Brumagne, Jean-Marie Caroyer, Joel Thimpont, Carine Sohy et al.** Occupational asthma in symptomatic workers exposed to natural rubber latex: Evaluation of diagnostic procedure. J Allergy Clin Immunol 2001; 107:542-7.

115. **Tee RD, Cullinan P, Welch J, Burge PS, Newman-Taylor AJ.** Specific IgE to isocyanates: a useful diagnostic role in occupational asthma. J Allergy Clin Immunol 1998; 101: 709-15.

116. **Jeremy Beach, MBBS, Kelly Russell, Sandra Blitz, Nicola Hooton, Carol Spooner et al.** A Systematic Review of the Diagnosis of Occupational Asthma. Chest 2007; 131; 569-78.

117. **V. Cottin.** Bronchite a eosinophiles Eosinophilic bronchitis. Revue fran^aise d'allergologie et d'immunologie clinique 2008; 48: 196-200.

118. **Fournier M, Couvelard A, Mal H, Groussard O.** Constrictive bronchiolitis in adults outside the context of transplantation. Revue des Maladies Respiratoires 2006; 23: 657-66.

119. **Thaon I, Reboux G, Moulonguet S, Dalphin J C.** Les pneumopathies d'hypersensibilite en milieu professionnel Occupational hypersensitivity pneumonitis. Revue des Maladies Respiratoires 2006; 23: 705-25.

120. **Bodenes A, Andre M, Dewitte J D, Quiot J J, Potard G, Mialon P et al.** Vocal cord dysfunction of occupational origin. Archives des Maladies Professionnelles et de l'Environnement 2002; 63: 87-90.

121. **Coppieters Y, Nemery B, Piette D.** Étude bibliographique de l'efficacite des actions de prévention de l'asthme professionnel. Sante publique 2003; 15: 423-35.

122. **Padoan M, Pozzato V, Simoni M, Zedda L, Milan G, Bononi I et al.** Longterm follow-up of toluene diisocyanate-induced asthma. European Respiratory Journal 2003; 21: 637-40.

123. **Vandenplas O, Toren K, Blanc P D.** Health and socioeconomic impact of work-related asthma. Eur Respir J 2003; 22: 689-97.

124. **Gianna Moscato, Antonio Dellabianca, Luca Perfetti, Barbara Brame, Eugenia Galdi, Rosanna Niniano et al.** Occupational Asthma: A Longitudinal Study on the Clinical and Socioeconomic Outcome After diagnosis. Chest 1999; 115: 249-56.

125. **Larbanois A, Jamart J, Delwiche J P, Vandenplas O.** Socioeconomic outcome of subjects experiencing asthma symptoms at work. Eur Respir J 2002; 19: 1107-13.

126. **Pauli G, Gonzalez M, Bessot J C.** Occupational asthma: what background treatment, what prevention? Is there a place for desensitisation? Archives des maladies professionnelles et de medecine du travail 2002; 63: 638-43.

127. **Jeremy Beach, Brian H Rowe, Sandra Blitz, Ellen Crumley, Nicola Hooton, Kelly Russell et al.** Diagnosis and Management of Work-Related Asthma. Evidence Report Technology Assessment 2005; 129: 1-8.

128. **Alessandra Marabini, Andrea Siracusa, Roberta Stopponi, Cinzia Tacconi, Giuseppe Abbritti.** Outcome of Occupational Asthma in Patients with Continuous Exposure: A 3-Year Longitudinal Study During Pharmacologic Treatment. Chest 2003; 124: 2372-6.

129. **A Marabini, H Dimich-Ward, S Y Kwan, S M Kennedy, N Waxler- Morrison, M Chan-Yeung.** Clinical and socioeconomic features of subjects with red cedar asthma. A follow-up study. Chest 1993; 104: 821-4.

130. **Malo J L, Cartier A, Cote J, Milot J, Leblanc C, Paquette L et al.** Influence of inhaled steroids on recovery from occupational asthma after cessation of exposure: an 18-month double-blind crossover study. Am. J. Respir. Crit. Care Med 1996; 153: 953-60.

131. **M. Ndiaye, J. Bousquet, H. Dhivert-Donnadieu, P. Godard, P. Demoly.** L'immunotherapie specifique dans la rhinite allergique et l'asthme: quand et comment l'instituer puis l'arreter? Rev Fr Allergol Immunol Clin 2002; 42: 324-9.

132. **Sastre Joaquin, Quirce Santiago.** Immunotherapy: an option in the management of occupational asthma? Current Opinion in Allergy & Clinical Immunology: 2006; 6: 96-100.

133. **Joaquin Sastre, Mar Fernandez-Nieto, Pilar Rico, Santiago Martin, Domingo Barber, Javier Cuesta et al.** Specific immunotherapy with a standardized latex extract in allergic workers: A double-blind, placebocontrolled Study. J Allergy Cl Fn Immunol 2003;

111: 986- 94.
134. **Ernesto Enrique, Fernando Pineda, Tamim Malek, Joan Bartra, Maria Basagan, Raquel Tella et al.** Sublingual immunotherapy for hazelnut food allergy: A randomized, double-blind, placebo-controlled study with a standardized hazelnut extract. J Allergy Clin Immunol 2005 ; 116: 1073-9.
135. **David D. Rutstein, Robert J. Mullan, Todd M. Frazier, William E. Halperin, James M. Melius, John P. Sestito.** Sentinel Health Events (Occupational): A Basis for Physician Recognition And Public Health Surveillance. AJPH 1983; 73, 1054-62.
136. **Baur X, Degens P, Weber K.** Occupational obsmactive airway diseases in Germany. Am J Ind Med 1998; 33: 454-62.
137. **Van de Weyer R.** Principes generaux de reparation et de prevention des maladies professionnelles respiratoires en Belgique. Rev Mal Resp 1990; 7: 126-34.
138. **Innocenti A.** Occupational asthma: considerations on epidemiology and criteria of damage evaluation. Med Lav. 1997; 88: 3-12.
139. **Kjell Toren.** Self reported rate of occupational asthma in Sweden 19901992. Occupational and Environmental Medicine 1996; 53:757-61.
140. **Walls C, Crane J, Gillies J, Wilsher M, Wong C.** Occupational asthma and other nonasbestos occupational respiratory diseases notified between 1993 and 1996. New Zealand Med J 1997; 110: 246-9.
141. **Ross DJ.** Ten years of the SWORD project. Clin Exp Allergy 1999 ; 29: 7503.
142. **Ameille J.** Asthme professionnel : Consequences socio-economiques et professionnelles de l'asthme professionnel. Rev Mal Respir 2000; 17: 284-7.
143. Order of the Ministries of Public Health and Social Affairs. Bareme indicatif des taux d'invalidite permanente resultant des accidents de travail et des maladies professionnelles. Journal officiel de la Republique Tunisienne N°26 31 mars 1995.
144. **Pauli G, Kopferschmitt-Kubler MC.** Medical prognosis. In: L'asthme professionnel, JC Bessot, G Pauli ; Eds Margaux Orange, Paris, 1999, 523535.
145. **Ameille J, Descatha A.** Outcome of occupational asthma. Curr Opin Allergy Clin Immunol 2005; 5: 125-8.
146. **Fabbri LM, Danieli D, Crescioli S, Bevilacqua P, Meli S, Saetta M, Mapp CE.** Fatal asthma in a subject sensitized to toluene diisocyanate. Am Rev Respir Dis 1998; 137: 1494-8.
147. **Coppieters Y, Nemery B, Piette D.** Etude bibliographique de l'efficacite des actions de prevention de l'asthme professionnel. Societe fran^aise de sante publique Sante publique 2003; 15: 423-35.
148. **Dewitte J D, Chan-Yeung M, Malo J L.** Medicolegal and compensation aspects of occupational asthma. Eur Respir J. 1994, 7, 969-980.
149. **Gonzalez M, Cantineau A, Bessot J C, Pauli G.** Collective and individual prevention. In: L'asthme professionnel. Eds Margaux Orange1999; 537-47.

Occupational asthma

I. Patient identity

1- Name :

2- First name :

3- Sex: 1- male; 2-female.

4- Age (year) :

5- File number :

6- Telephone number : ; address :

II. Socio-professional data

A- Origin :

1- urban 2-rural.

B- Marital status :

1- single2-marie (e)

3-divorce 4- widow(er)

C-School level :

1-literacy 2-primary education

3-Secondary education; 4-Higher education.

D-Professional category :

1-worker; 2-middle manager; 3-senior manager; 4-employee

E-Nature du regime social : (CNAM)

1-public; 2-prive; 3-indigent

F-Labour sector :

1- -agriculture -fishing ;

2- building and public works ;

3- Primary sector: heavy industry and mining

4- Secondary sector (Manufacturing industry)

5- Tertiary sector (services)

G-Company: ; address :

H-Profession :

J- Date of hire (years) :

K- seniority :

1- < 5years ; 2- [5years - 15years [; 3- [15years - 25years [; 4- >25years

L-Nature of the exhibition :

111.Background

A- Family history of atopy :

1- none; 2-asthma; 3-rhinitis; 4-conjunctivitis; 5-eczema; 6-other.

B-Personal history :

a) Atopic :

1- No

2- Asthma
3- Rhinitis
4- Conjunctivitis
5- Eczema

6- Other b) other

1-None
2-Tuberculosis
3-BPCO
4-DDB
5-Other

C- Genetic susceptibility :

1- HLA typing :
2- Genetic factor :

IV.Habits :

1- No
2- Tobacco a- pack/year
b- Duration
3- Neffa :
4- Narguile :
5- Alcohol: a- Chronic b- Occasional

V. Address by :

1- Occupational physician
2- Free-lance doctor
3- Hospital service
4- GMT/IMT
5- UGTT
6- CNAM
7- Other

VI.Reason for consultation :

1- notice of fitness (pre-recruitment visit, other)
2- confirmation of occupational illness
3- diagnostic opinion
4- PPI assessment
5- disability
6- notice for early retirement
7- other

VII. Diagnosis of asthma

A. Data from the interview :

a. Respiratory symptoms :

1- Wheezing dyspnea
2- Dry cough
3- Chest tightness
4- Shortness of breath on exertion
5- Chronic exertional dyspnea

b. Associated atopic symptoms :

1- No
2- Rhinitis
3- Conjunctivitis
4- skin lesions
5- Others.

B. Clinical assessment :

1- Normal
2- Sibilant rales
3- Buzzing Rales
4- Chest distension
5- Other

C. Paraclinical assessment

A/ Biology

a. NFS :

1- Not done
2- normal eosinophilia
3- hyper eosinophilia

b. Total IgE :

1- Not done
2- Standard rate
3- Rate Increases UI/ml

B/ Radiological assessment

a. Chest X-ray :

1- Not done
2- Normal
3-Normal (distension, emphysema bubbles, cardiomegaly, other)

b. sinus x-ray :

1- Not done
2- Normal
3- Abnormal

C/ Functional respiratory investigation (FRI)

1- Not done
2- Normal
3- Obstructive syndrome
4- Restrictive syndrome
5- Mixed syndrome

VEMS% CV% VEMS/CV

D/ Reversibility test :

1- Not done
2- Negative
3- Positive

E/ Non-specific bronchial provocation test :

1-Not done
2- Negative
3- Positive

F/ Standard patch test

1- Not done
2- Negative
3- positive

VIII. Asserting the occupational nature of asthma :

A- Examination data :

a- Delay in onset of symptoms in relation to work

1- Immediate
2- < 1 year
3- [1- 5 years [
4- [5-10 years [
5- [10-15 years [
6- [15-20 years [
7- >20 years

b-Chronology of symptoms :

1-Acurrence and aggravation during work and improvement during weekends and holidays.

2-Permanent.

3- Existing prior to recruitment.

8- Job study

a- 1-Done ; 2- Not done

b- Etiological agents involved

1. Chemical (isocyanate; anhydride; amine; rosin; formaldehyde; chloramine; persulphate; antibiotic; azabis formamide)
2. Metals (a-platinum; b-nickel; c-chromium; d-cobalt; e-galvanised steel, aluminium)
3. Animal: laboratory animals (a-rat; b-mouse; d-rabbit; e-pig); seafood (a-crab; b-shrimp); gum.
4. plant: flour (a- grain dust; b- wheat; c- rye; d- buckwheat; e- coffee beans; f- soya beans); red cedar; wood; latex.
5. Other

c- Handling conditions :

1- Closed vessel; 2- Gun; 3- Mask; 4- Other

d- Occupational health coverage :

1-yes2-no

e- Conclusion:

C- Allergological test :

a-Specific IgE (RAST)

1- Not done

2- Negative

3- - IncreaseUI /ml

b- -Specific skin test (specific prick test)

1- Not done

2- Negative

3- Positive

c- Specific bronchial provocation test: ...

1- Not done

2- Negative

3- Positive

4- Incidents Specify :

D. Debimetrie:

1- Outside work
2- At the exhibition
E. Staged spirometry :
1-Outside work :
VEMS.. . ; CV..VEMS/CV...
2-During the exhibition
VEMS.. . ; CV..VEMS/CV...
F. Eviction test :
1. Not done
2. Negative
3. positive

IX. Severity level :

1- Intermittent
2- Light evergreen
3- Moderate persistence
4- Persistent severe

X. Treatment

A- Eviction :
1-yes2-no
B-Pace of treatment :
1- Emergency treatment
2- Long-term background treatment C-Molecules :
1- Beta 2+ a action immediate inhale
2- Inhaled Beta 2+ long-acting
3- Beta 2+ long-acting oral
4- Long-acting oral euphylline
5- Low-dose inhaled corticoids
6- Inhaled corticoids medium dose

7- High-dose inhaled corticoids
8- Long-term oral corticoids
9- Nasal corticoids
10- Antihistamine
11- Anti leucotrienes.
12- Fixed combination beta 2+ corticoids
13- Free combination beta 2+ corticoids
14- Others.

XI. Medical and legal consequences

A-Declaration :

1 - Made date of declaration..."'..."'
2 - Not done
8- Table No. :
C- Etiological agent
D- Recognition as an occupational disease:...
1- Ouidate of recognition.../.../...
2- No
E- Repair :
1- no
2- PPI rate <= 4%.
3- PPI [5-14%] rate
4- PPI rate > 14
F- Reasons for rejection :
1-Medical
2-Administrative
3-Other :
G - Socio-professional consequences :
1- Retention in the same position
2- Job transfer
3- Reclassification
4- Dismissal.

XII. Evolution :

1-Total regression 2-Partial regression 3-Steady state or worsening.

A-Total eviction with symptomatic asthma for less than six months and no treatment :

8- Total exclusion with symptomatic asthma for less than six months and with treatment:

C- No eviction with symptomatic asthma of less than six months and with treatment

D-Total eviction with symptomatic asthma for more than six months and no treatment :

E- Total exclusion with symptomatic asthma for more than six months and with treatment:

F- No eviction with symptomatic asthma for more than six months and with treatment

XIII. Complication:

1- No

2- Yes ; Please specify :

Resume

Problems :

Occupational asthma (OA) has become the most common work-related respiratory disease. Moreover, epidemiological data suggest that 10% of adult asthma can be attributed to occupational activity. This disease affects a young, economically active population, and thus has a considerable socio-economic cost.

Aim of the work:

To study the prevalence of PA in southern Tunisia from 2002 to 2009, to establish its diagnostic strategy, to describe the epidemiological features of the subjects affected, the etiological factors and to specify the therapeutic, evolutionary, preventive and medico-legal aspects of the disease.

Materials and methods :

We carried out a retrospective descriptive study of all cases of PA declared to the regional offices of the CNAM over an eight-year period from 01/01/2002 to 31/12/2009, with the following objectives We collected data from the medical records used to establish the diagnosis of bronchial asthma, the medical and administrative records of patients declared for PA collected from the regional offices of the CNAM in Sfax, as well as the reports of the occupational survey carried out for all declared cases.

Results:

Fifty-nine cases of PA were collected in our study, with a mean age of 42+/9 years. The population was predominantly male. Most of the patients reported were manual workers employed by companies in the secondary sector.

Once the diagnosis of PA has been established, the treating physician, in collaboration with the occupational physician, proceeds with the declaration. In the context of our study, this was done essentially under 3 tables: table No. 42 relating to isocyanates; table No. 56 relating to cereals and flour; table No. 58: corresponding to other agents responsible for allergic respiratory diseases.

Of the 59 cases reported, 38 were recognised as occupational diseases. A rate of permanent partial disability was assigned to each recognised case (average permanent partial disability was 24.07%).

Twenty patients experienced a deterioration in their respiratory condition, requiring treatment and regular monitoring, while fifteen patients lost their jobs.

Conclusion:

PA is one of the most common occupational diseases, but it is often underestimated and/or under-reported. Given the potential seriousness of its socio-medical consequences, it is imperative to optimise its management in terms of both prevention and treatment.

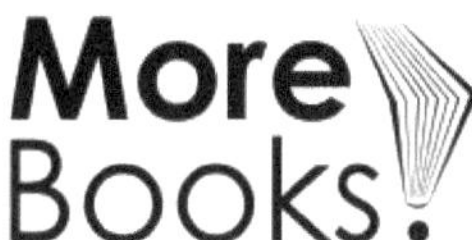

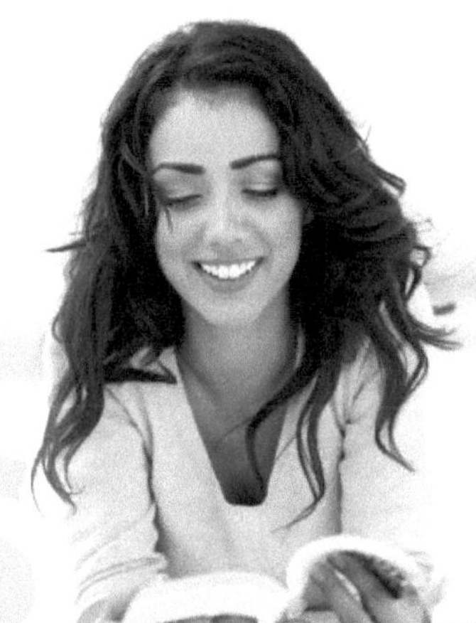

I **want** morebooks!

Buy your books fast and straightforward online - at one of world's fastest growing online book stores! Environmentally sound due to Print-on-Demand technologies.

Buy your books online at
www.morebooks.shop

Kaufen Sie Ihre Bücher schnell und unkompliziert online – auf einer der am schnellsten wachsenden Buchhandelsplattformen weltweit! Dank Print-On-Demand umwelt- und ressourcenschonend produzi ert.

Bücher schneller online kaufen
www.morebooks.shop

info@omniscriptum.com
www.omniscriptum.com

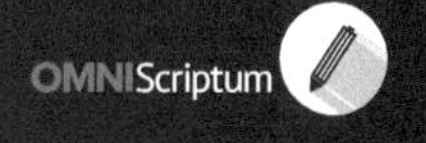

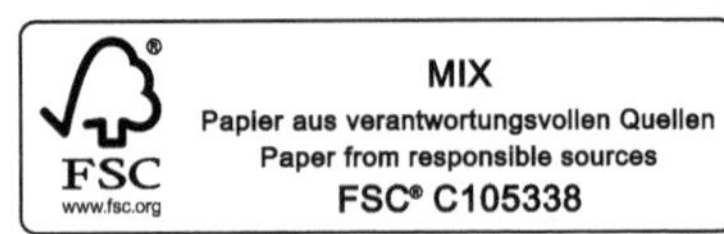

Printed by Books on Demand GmbH, Norderstedt / Germany